Introduction

This book is a reference and illustrated guide to the major organs of the human body. I continue to receive suggestions and feedback in reference to these books and I cannot stress how valuable these are to me. I feel with each book a new level is reached and this is due to constant vigilance. You, who write to me, shape the order of future titles and change the format of the books, so please keep this up!!! It is hoped this book will form another valuable chapter in the A to Z story. Human mechanics is a beautiful thing.

The A to Zs may be viewed on 2 sites –

www.amandasatoz.com and http://www.aspenpharma.com.au/atlas/student.htm

Feedback may be left at

anatomy.update@gmail.com / medicalamanda@gmail.com

and it is always appreciated.

Acknowledgement

Thank you Aspenpharmacare Australia for your support and assistance in this valuable project, particularly Mr. Greg Lan, CEO of Aspenpharmacare Australia, Rob Koster and Richard Clement.

Dedication

To those who – don't lock themselves in; those not goal orientated but life orientated and to Paul who did not live to see all of 2013 but who did live every moment. I wish I had dedicated a book to him before it was too late. To whom will I give my 1st A to Z now?

How to use this book

The format of this A to Z book has been maintained. The first section - The Cell lists the cell's major organelles, processes & types in the A to Z way. The second section lists the major organs. So as usual **think of it and then find it** is the motto of **the A to Zs** and continues to be the structure behind the book. How are the major organs considered? First as an organ as a whole; a macroscopic structure, then as a group of organized cells, an histological view and then as a machine doing a specific task, where it is illustrated as a schema. This subject is so large that it was not possible to include everything – good editing cannot be over-rated. So the reproductive organs have been omitted and will be dealt with in their own A to Z, and additional information may found in *the A to Z of the Brain and Cranial Nerves*, **the A to Z of the Heart**, *the A to Z of the Digestive Tract*, and *the A to Z of Hair, Nails & Skin* in particular, but as with all **the A to Zs** this book is complete unto itself.

Thank you

Amanda Neill
BSc MSc MBBS PhD FACBS
ISBN 9781921930065

T0319296

© A. L. Neill

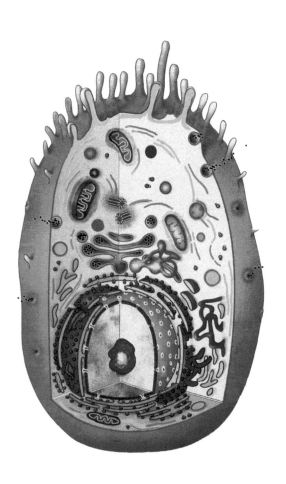

TABLE OF CONTENTS

THE CELL

THE ORGANS

Abbreviations

a	= artery	**Cr**	= cranial
aa	= anastomosis (ses)	**CT**	= connective tissue
AA	= amino acid	**CVS**	= cardiovascular system
Ab	= antibody	**DCT**	= distal convoluted tubules
ACTH	= adrenocorticotropic hormone / adrenal cortical hormone	**DNA**	= deoxyribonucleic acid
ADH	= antidiuretic hormone	**DT**	= digestive tract
adj.	= adjective	**diff.**	= difference(s)
ADP	= adenosine diphosphate	**dist.**	= distal
Ag	= antigen	**DM**	= dura mater
AKA	= also known as	**DT**	= digestive tract
alt.	= alternative	**E**	= energy
AMP	= adenosine monophosphate	**e.g.**	= example
ANS	= autonomic nervous system	**EAM**	= external acoustic meatus
ant.	= anterior	**EAS**	= external anal sphincter
AS	= Alternative Spelling, generally referring to the diff. b/n British & American spelling	**ec**	= extracellular (outside the cell)
		ext.	= extensor (as in muscle to extend across a joint)
ATP	= adenosine triphosphate	**GA**	= Golgi apparatus
B	= blood	**GALT**	= gut associated lymphoid tissue
bb	= basal bodies	**GB**	= gall bladder
bc	= because	**GH**	= growth hormone
BF	= blood flow	**GIT**	= gastro-intestinal tract
BM	= basement membrane / basal lamina / terminal lamina	**Gk.**	= Greek
		GM	= grey matter
b/n	= between	**gld**	= gland
BP	= blood pressure	**H**	= hormone
br	= branch	**H&E**	= haematoxylin & eosin
BS	= Blood Supply	**HP**	= high pressure
CC	= cerebral cortex	**IAM**	= internal acoustic meatus
c.f.	= compared to	**IAS**	= internal anal sphincter
CH	= cerebral henispheres	**ic**	= intracellular (inside the cell)
CL	= corpus luteum	**Jc**	= junctional complex
CM	= cellular membrane / plasma membrane	**jt(s)**	= joints = articulations
		L	= lumbar / left
CN	= cranial nerve	**L&R**	= left and right
CNS	= central nervous system	**LI**	= large intestine
CO	= cardiac output	**lig**	= ligament
Co	= coccygeal	**LP**	= lamina propria
CP	= cervical plexus	**LT**	= lymphoid tissue
collat.	= collateral	**Lt.**	= Latin

LIF	=	left iliac fossa
LP	=	lamina propria
LUQ	=	left upper quadrant
LV	=	left ventricle
m	=	muscle
med.	=	medial
mem	=	membrane
mito	=	mitochondrium (a)
mm	=	mucus membrane
m-RNA	=	messenger RNA
mv	=	microvillus (i)
N (s)	=	nerve(s)
NAD	=	normal (size, shape)
NAD	=	no abnormality detected
NM	=	nuclear membrane / nucleolemma
NR	=	nerve root origin
NS	=	nerve supply / nervous system
NT	=	nervous tissue
nv	=	neurovascular bundle
PAS	=	periodic acid-schiff stain
PCT	=	proximal convoluted tubules
pl.	=	plural
PN	=	peripheral nerve
post.	=	posterior
proc.	=	process
prox.	=	proximal
RA	=	right atrium
R	=	right / resistance
RIF	=	right iliac fossa
RNA	=	ribonucleic acid
rRNA	=	ribosomal RNA
RUQ	=	right upper quadrant
RV	=	right ventricle
SC	=	spinal cord
SI	=	small intestine
sing.	=	singular
SN	=	spinal nerve
SP	=	sacral plexus
SS	=	signs and symptoms

subcut.	=	subcutaneous (just under the skin)
supf	=	superficial
SVC	=	superior vena cava
T	=	thoracic / tissue
T3	=	tri-iodothyronine
T4	=	thyroxine
TNF	=	tumour necrosis factor
t-RNA	=	transfer RNA / transport RNA
TSH	=	thyroid stimulating hormone / thyrotropic hormone
tw	=	terminal web
V	=	vein
v	=	very
WM	=	white matter
w/n	=	within
w/o	=	without
wrt	=	with respect to
ZA	=	zonula adherens
ZO	=	zonula occludens / tight junction
&	=	and
∩	=	intersection with

Common terms used to describe Organs

A

Adenoid glandular

Alveolus air filled cavity e.g. tooth socket *adj. alveolar* (as in air filled bone in the Maxilla).

Anions negatively charged atoms or radicals e.g. C1⁻, OH⁻

Annulus fibrosis the peripheral fibrous ring around the intervertebral disc.

Aperture an opening or space between bones or within a bone.

Apocrine secretions which take off the cytoplasm of the apex of the cell as well

Areola small, open spaces as in the areolar part of the Maxilla may lead or develop into sinuses.

Arytenoid ladle or pitcher (arytenoid cartilages move in and out like ladle with changing sounds).

Atrium waiting room,

Attrition tooth wear and tear.

Autocrine secretions of the cell influence other like cells and its own function.

Autophagy the digestion of organelles (1) and other internal structures (2) or substances (3) by the cell itself via lysosomes (4). If the particles are large *Macroautophagy* they must first be internalized by ER (5) before they fuse with the lysosome (6)- otherwise as with smaller proteins - they are directly incorporated into the lysosome (7) - *Microautophagy* or have a "chaperone" protein (8) which transports them to the lysosome.

Axial refers to the head and trunk (vertebrae, ribs and sternum) of the body.

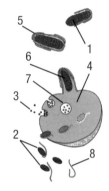

B

Biogenesis the development or formation of... e.g. biogenesis of an organelle may result from the fusion of several components ± their further modification.

Buccal *(BUK-al)* pertaining to the cheek.

C

Canal tunnel / extended foramen as in the carotid canal at the base of the skull *adj. canular* (canicule - small canal).

Cataract *(KAT-ar-akt)* opacity of the lens in the eye - may occur in the centre - nuclear, under the capsule subcapsular or in the cortex cortical.

Cations positively charged atoms or radicals e.g. NAD^+, Na^+, H^+, Ca^{++}

Caput / Kaput the head or of a head, *adj. capitate = having a head (c.f. decapitate)*

Capitus AKA Capitus* *adj. pertaining to the Head.*

Caveolin membrane-bound proteins involved in receptor-dependant endocytosis *pl. caveolae.*

Cavity an open area or sinus w/n a bone or formed by two or more bones *(adj. cavernous)* may be used interchangeably with fossa. Cavity tends to be more enclosed fossa a shallower bowl like space (Orbital fossa-Orbital cavity).

Cephalic pertaining to the head.

Cervicus AKA Cervicis* *adj. pertaining to the neck*

Clara cells "clear and famous" cells - the bulging cells seen in bronchioles which function as stem cells and replace the lining and alveolar cells. These cells produce surfactant and $\downarrow$ the surface tension on the surface of the alveoli and ease the entrance of the air.

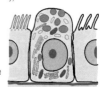

Codon a series of 3 nucleic bases which "code for the attachment of a particular AA in the synthesis of a protein - part of the the genetic code - note that the code for AAs in the mitochondria vary from "the genetic code".

Colon term used interchangeably with LI but actually only consisting of 4 parts - the ascending + transverse + descending + sigmoid colons – not including the caecum or appendix.

Concha *(KONG-ku)* a shell shaped bone as in the ear or nose *(pl. conchae adj. chonchoid)* old term for this turbinate.

Constrictor to squeeze - generally referring to a muscle's action where it decreases the size of an opening (as in Pharynx), different from sphincter, it does not stop the passage of a substance just modifies it.

Convoluted twisted and turning as in the renal tubules.

Cornu a horn (as in the Hyoid).

Corona a crown. *adj. coronary, coronoid or coronal*; hence a coronal plane is parallel to the main arch of a crown which passes from ear to ear *(c.f. coronal suture).*

Cranium the cranium of the skull comprises all of the bones of the skull except for the mandible.

Crest prominent sharp thin ridge of bone formed by the attachment of muscles particularly powerful ones e.g. Temporalis/Sagittal crest.

Cribiform / Ethmoid a sieve or bone with small sieve-like hole

Cricoid a ring

-crine to secrete

Cutus *(KEW-tis)* skin - *adj. cutaneous* it has come to refer only to the epidermis.

D

Dens a tooth, denticulate having tooth-like projections *adj. dental, dentate, dentine denticulate.*

Dentine (AKA) dentin ivory–like substance forming the bulk of the tooth beneath the enamel.

Depression a concavity on a surface.

Dermis the CT of skin

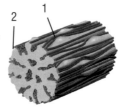

Desquamated the shedding of keratinized layer of the skin *see also exfoliated.*

Distal further away from the axial skeleton *(opposite to Proximal)* in dentistry = along the dental arch in posterior direction (opposite to Mesial).

Dorsi back. *adj. dorsal*

E

Edentulous w/o teeth.

Elastin major extracellular fibre which has recoil properties - made up of fibrillin (1) filaments and elastin matrix (2) which assemble from smaller ic components outside the cell.

endo- into

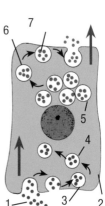

Endocrine secretion of a substance from cells directly to the BS w/o a duct *(opposite of Exocrine).*

Endocytosis is the major form of vesicular transport in the cell - material (1) such as small proteins attach to the CM (2) which invaginates & encloses it disconnecting from the CM (3) forming a vesicle (4) *see also Exocytosis* as pictured.

Endosomes membrane-bound body in the cell generally from ingested material and requiring further digestion – a progression in the path to lysosome differentiation *see also Lysosome, Vesicle.*

exo- out of

Exocrine secretion of substances from cells onto a surface or lumen possibly via ducts as in exocrine glands generally into a lumen, but maybe on a surface *(≠ Endocrine).*

Exocytosis is the major form of vesicular transport - vesicles in the cell (5) move from their site to the CM (6) attaching to the surface (7) and then fusing with it to release the contents *see also Endocytosis* as pictured.

External Auditory Meatus ear hole = EAM.

extra- outside of

F

Facet *(FASS-et)* a face, a small bony surface (occlusal facet on the chewing surfaces of the teeth) seen in planar joints.

Fascia *(FASH-uh)* face / layers of CT.

Fascicle *(FAS-ik-el)* small bundle.

Fauces *(FOR-seez)* jaws or throat.

Fibril a small fibre or filament at least 10X smaller than the main type of fibrous structure and a smaller part of a larger structure as in myofibril.

Filament a single thread or strand which may be thick or thin but is not made up of obvious multiple units as may be the case in a fibre.

Fibre ASA fiber *see also Filament* a rope or long strand of material - may have multiple monomeric units joined together or filaments woven together in its makeup and appear as a single unit in biology there are 4 main types - the collagens; the elastins, the fibrillins and the fibronectins, but the most important by far is the collagen group *adj. fibrillar.*

Fissure *(FISH-er)* a narrow slit or gap from cleft.

Flexure a fixed bend generally due to a tether by lig. or mesentery to the peritoneal wall as in the Hepatic flexure of the LI.

Foramen a natural hole in a bone usually for the transmission of BVs &/or Ns. *(pl. foramina).*

Fossa a pit, depression, or concavity, on a bone, or formed from several bones as in temporomandibular fossa - shallower and more like a "bowl" than a cavity.

Fovea *(FOH-vee-ar)* a small pit (usually smaller than a fossa) - as in the fovea of the occlusal surface of the molar tooth.

Free radicals unbound charged ions or molecules - highly reactive *see also Radicals.*

G

GALT a general term for all the lymphoid tissue associated with the GIT.

Gastric belly (as in the belly of a muscle).

Gingiva gum.

Gland epithelial cells which secrete material that has an effect on other cells.

Glottis pertaining to the vocal cords and structures involved in the production of the voice *pl. glottedis.*

Glycan a sugar.

Glycosylation attachment of 1 or more sugars to a molecule.

Gomphosis *(GOM-foh-sis)* joint b/n the roots of the teeth and the jaw bones *pl. gomphoses.*

Groove long pit or furrow.

H

H&E routine stain used in histology - demonstrates most organelles based on their affinity for acid & bases in contrasting blue (staining basophilic or acid substances) & pink (strongly staining bases or acidophilic substances) colours.

Haematochezia bright red clots of blood in the stools.

Haem (AS Heme) chemical compound consisting of iron ion in the centre of a large orgnanic ring.

Haematoxylin ASA Hematoxylin a dye extracted from the logwood tree; oxidised it forms haematein, a blue coloured commplex with metal ions notibly cell nuclei.

Hamus a hook hence the term used for bones which "hook around other bones or where other structures are able to attach by hooking - hamulus = a small hook.

Hepatomegaly enlargement of the liver

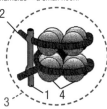

Histone an alkaline hydrophilic protein(1) used to organize the long DNA string (2) into structural units   nucelosomes (3), by coiling them around the 8 unit histone core (4) structure shortening he average 1.8m of DNA strand to 90µm. Active genes are less bound up in the histone core than inactive genes and they play a role in gene expression and suppression *see also Nucleosome.*

Holocrine secretions which involve the death of the cell with substance liberation.

Homeostasis *(HOH-me-oh-stay-sis)* condition of cells in organs or tissues where loss of the units (cells usually) is equal to the formation of new units A - most disease states can be simplified to belong to an inequality b/n cell proliferation & loss either ↑ in loss as in atrophy B or ↑ in proliferation as in cancer **C**

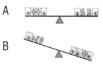

Hormones substances secreted by endocrine glands.

Hyoid U-shaped.

I

Incisura a notch

Incus anvil

Inferior under

Inter between *adj. intercalated*

Intercalated - e.g. intercalated discs or ducts inserted b/n other structures.

Intra within

Introitus an orifice or point of entry to a cavity or space.

Ions - charged atoms *see also Free Radicals*

   -- ve charge - anions - generally non-metal

   + ve charge - cations generally metal

L

Labia pertaining to the lips *(adj. labial)* may be oral or vulval lips.

Lacerum something lacerated, mangled or torn e.g. foramen lacerum small sharp hole at the base of the skull often ripping tissue in trauma.

Lacrima *(LAK-rim-u)* related to tears and tear drops *(adj. lacrimal)*.

Lambda *(LAM-duh)* from the Greek letter a capital 'L' and written as an inverted V *(adj. lambdoid)* and used to name the point of connection between the 3 skull bones Occiput and the 2 Temporal bones.

Lamina a plate or layer as in the lamina of the vertebra a plate of bone connecting the vertical and transverse spines *(pl. laminae)*.

Lamina propria (LP) proper layer, background T surrounding major specialized cell masses in an organ - often loose areolar T: a combination of CT, immune cells, BVs, lymphocytes & Ns.

Lens the solid structure in the eye which focuses the incident light contains capsule cortex and nucleus - the hardening of the nucleus is primarily responsible for presbyopia.

Levator to raise - generally in reference to the actions of muscles.

Ligament a band of tissue which connects bones (articular ligaments) or viscera - organs (visceral ligaments). A ligament is a tie or a connection originally *sing. ligamentum pl. ligamenta* from ligate or to tie up generally composed of collagen fibres.

Ligand a small molecule, that forms a complex with a biomolecule to serve a biological purpose. Often used as a signal triggering molecule, binding to a protein which alters its shape to allow attachment of another protein often an H.

Linea *(lin-EE-uh)* a line as in the Nuchal lines of the Occipitum.

Lingual *(ling-GEW-al)* pertaining to the tongue.

Lipofuscin protein which accumulates in a cell with age, related to the breakdown of fats &/or proteins.

Lymph *(LIMpf)* excess fluid & proteins left behind from the capillaries as they move from the arterial to the venous side.

M

macro- large

Malar cheek

Malleus hammer (as in the ear ossicle).

Mandible from the verb to chew, hence, the movable lower jaw; *adj. mandibular*.

Masseter to chew

Maxilla the jaw-bone; now used only for the upper jaw; *adj. maxillary*.

Meatus a short passage; *adj. meatal* as in external acoustic meatus connecting the outer ear with the middle ear.

Meibum an oily secretion from the Meibomian glds (AKA tarsal glds) of the eye to lubricate the cornea.

megaly- enlargement

Meiosis *(MY-oh-sis)* germ cell division where the genetic material is halved as a device for future fertilization.

Mental relating to the chin (mentum = chin *not mens = mind*).

Merocrine secretions which are due to exocytosis.

Mesial along the dental arch in the direction of the medial plane anteriorly (opposite to Distal).

micro- small pertaining to structures which are able to be viewed under the microscope.

Molecule a neutral group of atoms held together by ionic or covalent bonds - however it is often also a term used for a charged polyatomic group which are technically *Radicals*.

Monomers individual units of a larger structure - usually with the building up of extracellular fibres e.g. collagen *see also Polymers.*

Mucosa *(MEW-koh-zuh)* tissue in the GIT immediately beneath the epithelial lining.

Mucous *adj. of mucus* as in mucous glands – glands which produce mucus.

Mucus *(MEW-kus)* substance excreted by Mucous glands to lubricate food or protect mucosal surfaces.

Muscularis Mucosa (mm) term for the muscle layer in the mucosa separating the mucosa from the submucosa.

N

Naris nostrils *pl. Nares*

Notch an indentation in the margin of a structure.

Nucha the nape or back of the neck *adj. nuchal.*

Nucleolus *(NEWK-lee-oh-lus)* a small unbound collection of RNA w/n the nucleus which varies in size, shape and presence due to the activity of the cell. It is the site of rRNA synthesis and dispersement, and the assembly of ribosomes. It appears as a darkly staining spot(s) in the nucleus *pl. nucleoli*

Nucleosome a coil of DNA wrapped around a histone core as a form of organized packing *see also Histone.*

O

Occiput the prominent convexity of the back of the head Occipitum = Occipital bone *adj. occipital.*

Occlusion opposition of the teeth when closed = bite.

Orbit a circle; the name given to the bony socket in which the eyeball rotates; *adj.orbital.*

ORGAN - A GROUP OF TISSUES & CELLS WHICH ARE BOUND TOGETHER TO PERFORM A SPECIFIC FUNCTION.

Orifice *(or-EE-fiss)* an opening.

Ossicle small bone – generally referring to the bones in the ear.

P

Palate a roof *adj. palatal or palatine.*

Papilla (e) outpouching – point generally with an opening (c.f. the duodenal papilla.)

Paracrine substances secreted which only have local effects - as in the pilo-sebacious unit hair follicle.

Parenchyma *(PA-ren-KY-muh)* main component of an organ when it is highly cellular e.g. the liver.

Parietal *(pa-RYE-et-al)* pertaining to the outer wall of a cavity from paries, a wall.

Parotid *(pa-ROT-id)* pertaining to a region beside or near the ear.

Pars a part of

Peri- around surrounding

Perikymata transverse ridges and the grooves on the surfaces of teeth.

Periodontum CT membrane surrounding the tooth to allow for support and cushioning of tooth movements with mastication.

Periosteum layer of fascial tissue connective tissue on the outside of compact bone not present on articular (joint) surfaces *see endostium.*

Peristalsis the automatic coordinated contraction & relaxation of the GIT smooth muscle triggered by the presence of a food bolus & propagated by the internal NS of the GIT the Auerbach & Myenteric plexi – directing food in one direction.

Peroxisome vesicles .2-.5µm containing dense particle involved in the catabolism of fatty acids and the synthesis of plasma proteins & cholesterol. They contain relevant enzymes to help in this process and are commonest in hepatocytes and only have a sinle lipid layer - different from most ic membrane bound vesicles.

Petrous pertaining to a rock / rocky / stony *adj. petrosal*

phago *(FAY-goh)* **to eat**

Phagocytosis the active ingestion of larger particles and their digestion and inactivation w/n the cell.

Phosphorylation addition of 1 or more phophate radicals to a structure - usually protein

pilo- hair

Pinocytosis *(pyn-OH-sy-toh-sis)* the dynamic formation of small vesicles (1) endosomes (2) in the cell to ingest material (3) *adj. pinocytic.*

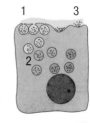

Plasma is blood w/o its cellular components *see also Serum*

Plica (e) *(PLEE-ku/kay)* fold (s) generally fixed folds with a CT stem to fix their shape – cannot be flattened as in SI.

Polymers repeated "monomer" units as in several monomers of the collagen fibre placed together but not enough to be a complete fibre *see also Monomer.*

Presbyopia *(PREZ-by-oh-pee-uh)* shortsightedness associated with age - inability to focus on close items.

Process a general term describing any marked projection or prominence as in the mandibular process.

Proximal closer to the axial skeleton *(opposite to Distal).*

Pseudophakic implanted prosthetic lens in the eye (generally due to cataracts).

R

Radicals charged atomic particles or charged polyatomic groups which may be bound to larger molecules or freely disassociated and "unbound"- *free radicals* - refer to an unbound charged ions or molecules - and are highly reactive.

Raphe *(RAF-ay)* line of joint b/n 2 halves, generally of bone or muscles for example a fibrous raphe in the tongue allowing for muscle insertion.

Recess a secluded area or pocket; a small cavity set apart from a main cavity.

Rectus straight, erect

Refered pain AKA reflected pain pain perceived in a different location from its site of origin.

Rhinus/rhino- *(RYE-noh)* pertaining to the nose.

Ridge elevated bony growth often roughened.

Rima Glottidis space b/n the vocal cords.

Rostral towards the anterior/front (of the brain).

Rotundum round

Ruga (e) *(ROO-gu/ gay)* folds – generally more mobile and less structured than Plicae – can be flattened as in the Stomach.

S

Sagittal *(SAJ-it-tal)* an arrow, the sagittal suture is notched posteriorly, making it look like an arrow by the lambdoid sutures.

Sclersosis hardening *adj sclerotic*

Senescence signs associated with aging e.g. in a cell the accumulation of lipofuscin is related to age.

Septum a division

Serum (blood) is blood plasma w/o the clotting factors i.e. it is acellular fluid with fewer proteins and cannot clot.

Sinus a space usually w/in a bone lined with mm, such as the frontal & maxillary sinuses in the head, (also, a modified BV usually vein with an enlarged lumen for blood storage & containing no or little muscle in its wall). Sinuses may contain air, blood, lymph, pus or serous fluid depending upon location and health of the subject *adj. sinusoid.*

Skull the skull refers to all of the bones that comprise the head.

Spine a thorn *adj. - spinous* descriptive of a sharp, slender process/protrusion commonly used regarding the spinous processes of the vertebral bodies.

Sphincter ring of muscle around a tube or opening, generally but not always, composed of skeletal muscle. generaly used to prevent the passage of a substance.

splanchno- *(SPLANK-noh)* **pertaining to the gut**

Splanchnocranium the splanchnocranium refers to the facial bones of the skull.

Splenomegaly - enlargement of the spleen.

-stoma to do with the mouth

Stroma *(STROH-mu)* underlying T background may have various structures but is often equivalent to lamina propria (LP).

sub- under

Subcutaneous under the skin, but has come to mean dermal - ie subepithelial.

Submucosa layer common to all the parts of the DT deep to the mucosa.

Sulcus long wide groove often due to a BV indentation.

Suture the saw-like edge of a cranial bone that serves as joint b/n bones of the skull.

Sulcus (i) *(SUL-kus/kee)* furrow cf in the brain

Superior above

syn- *(SIN)* **together i.e. the close proximity of or fusion of 2 structures**

T

Telomere end piece of the chromosome arms (1) which stabilizes the chromosome (2). If this is removed the cell becomes unstable and apoptosis may ensue; shortening is linked to senescence.

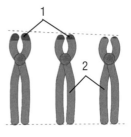

Temporal refers to time and the fact that grey hair (marking the passage of time) often appears first at the site of the temporal bone from the consideration of wisdom in the temple.

Tendon a tie or cord of collagen fibres connecting muscle with bone (as opposed to articular ligaments which connect bone with bone).

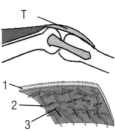

Tensor to stretch - generally referring to the action of a muscle which pulls something tighter.

Terminal web - fibrillar roof just beneath the CM (1) of epithelial cells composed of actin fibrils (2) & their links (3) to give structure to the cell surface, present in most epithelial cells.

Throat *(THROHT)* common term for pharynx and may incorporate the larynx as well as in sore throat

Tonsil little pole

Trachea *(TRAK-ee-uh)* rough

Transverse to go across.

Tuberosity a large rounded process or eminence, a swelling or large rough prominence often associated with a tendon or ligament attachment.

Tubules small tubes.

Turbinate a child's spinning top, hence shaped like a top; an old term for the nasal conchae.

U

Uvea *(YOU-vee-uh)* the combination of the iris + ciliary body + choroid plexus as a single entity - the BF b/n these 3 structures is continuous and so any pathology teds to involve all 3 at the same time.

Uvula *(YOUV-you-luh)* little grape

V

Vagina *(vaj-EYE-nuh)* a sheath; hence, invagination is the acquisition of a sheath by pushing inwards into a structure, and evagination is similar but produced by pushing outwards *adj. vaginal.*

Vertebra turning point.

Vesicle *(VEEZ-ik-el)* any membrane enclosed bubble w/n a cell - generally with the same bilipid layered as the CM and so it is possible for the vesicle to generate a separate internal environment w/n the cell - the cell's organelles are forms of vesicles.

W

Wormian bone extrasutural bone in the skull.

X

xero- *(ZAIR-oh)* **dry**

Xerostoma dry mouth

The Cell Membrane - CM

Micro Schema

The CM is a bilipid layer with protein insertions to facilitate transport in & out of the cell. It separates intracellular (ic) from extracellular (ec) environments by repelling hydrophilic substances. Because of its lipid nature, a charge maybe mounted across the CM and this is used in neural and contractile tissues, to communicate and initiate contractions. Proteins of the CM are integral proteins, but w/n this category there are a number of specialized forms. W/n the cell, organelles have their own membranes which have a similar basic structure, with their own controls and special adaptations.

1   single lipid layer

   e = external proteins – used to attract – or secure substances to the cell and activate their internalization

   i = internal proteins

   t = transmembrane proteins – used for protein transport

2   lipid bilayer = CM

3   hydrocarbon chain

4   hydrophilic head of the lipid chain – to allow the cell to remain in a "watery" environment

5   glycans and/or other sugars often with Ag properties

6   cholesterol insertions of the CM

7   plane of weakness in the CM – allows for shearing

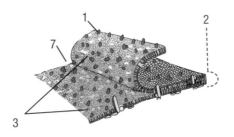

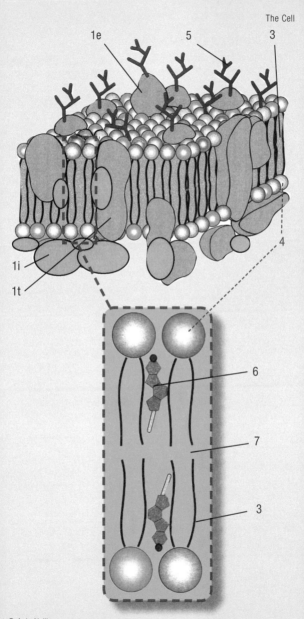

The Cell

1e

5

3

1i

1t

4

6

7

3

© A. L. Neill

21

The Cell Membrane - CM
Integral Proteins

Schema

Integral proteins are inserted into the CM, if they cross the whole CM, they are transmembranous proteins. As well as facilitating most transport across the CM - except for simple diffusion of lipid or fat materials, they perform a number of other functions.

1. CM
2. structural transmembrane proteins
3. enzyme proteins - substances pass through and emerge changed - having been in some form "digested"
4. linking proteins - bind fibrils to the CM on 1 or 2 sides; some do not go completely through the CM
5. actin - internal filaments
6. collagen - external fibres
7. receptor proteins - shaped to receive specific substances and move them from one to the other side of the CM (II)
8. Ca^{++} channel protein pump - composed of 6 subunits which open to allow the rapid influx/outflux of ions and changing the electrical charge of the CM (III).
9. Na^+/K^+ pump - constantly working to restore the CM charge - &/or coupling with other ions or charged radicals to facilitate their transport for ions to rapidly change the charge across the CM /or an internal membrane

I. simple diffusion - needs no protein to pass through the CM - hydrophobic substances only

II. facilitated transport via carrier proteins - receptor transport via protein channel if the substance is altered in the transport then this is enzymatic transport

III. rapid channel transport - mainly seen in contractile or neural tissue

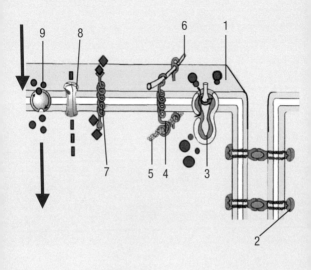

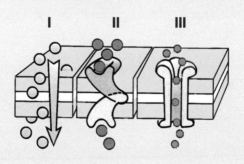

Centromeres

Schema

centromere structure overview

centromeres in mitosis

The centromeres of the cell have several roles. They organize the intracellular fibrils; their placements, attachments and pathways. aligning the chromatin, in mitosis, for the exchange of material, via the astral microtubules. They produce the bbs of cilia & flagellae, and contribute to the organization of the tw. They also play a role in the motility of the cell, and possibly its aging.

1 microtubule + ve end growing towards the CM
2 microtubules & filaments
       a = astral microtubules (starlike)
       k = kinetochore - kinetic - helping to separate and orientate the genes
       p = polar microtubules - upper & lowermost to help divide the cytoplasm in mitosis
3 NBBC = nucleus-basal body connector
4 nucleolus
5 nucleus
6 nuclear mem + ER + Golgi network
7 centromeres - note always at right angles to each other
8 MTOC = microtubule organizing centre - with growing bbs
9 cellular DNA genes

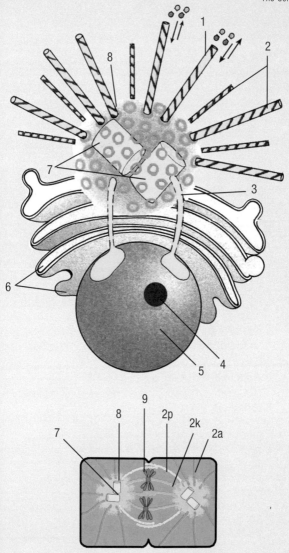

Chromatin

Schema

Packaging of DNA - and formation of chromatin and chromosomes

Chromatin is the language of the nucleus in the cell. It is formed by DNA which consists of molecular bases bound on a protein string arranged in tri-base codes. The actions of the cell are guided by the interpretation of these bases. Therefore the long strands of DNA must be organized and stored in a fashion that allows for appropriate retrieval so they are coiled & coiled & coiled... Primarily the DNA strands are wrapped around histone cores which are tightly bound in the inactive genes. These nucleosomes are then packed up into tightly coiled regions, further reducing the length. These packages form a region on a chromosome which may be further coiled in the mitosing cell.

1. DNA helix -   2nm wide
2. nucleosome beads -   11nm wide
   composed of histone core & lock and wrapped strands of DNA
3. nucleosome packing -   30nm wide
   composed of different groups of nucleosomes of related functions
4. extended chromosome -   300 nm wide
   containing several genes which may be made up of one or more of the nucleosome packages
5. coiled chromosome in active cell - 700nm wide
6. supercoiled chromosome -   1500nm wide
   during the mitotic process the chromosomes are further coiled along the microtubules & filaments

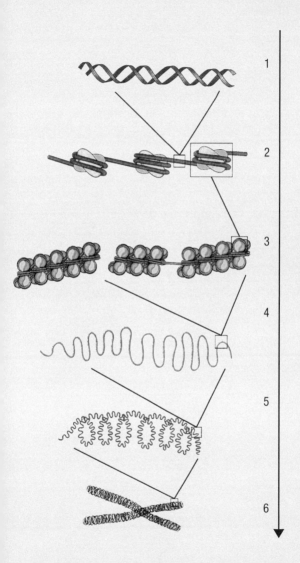

1

2

3

4

5

6

© A. L. Neill

Collagen

The collagens are a large family of proteins and have many different forms. They comprise the most important of the 4 fibrillar extracellular matrix components (collagen, elastin, fibrin & fibronectin). Fibrocytes synthesize most collagen but it can be synthesized by many cell types. Within the cell α chains are synthesized and they form triple helices = procollagen, which cannot bond into long fibrils. This is then extruded from the cell, where further modification allows long banded fibrils = tropocollagen. Further thickening and X-linking form collagen fibres, which develop in specific ways depending upon their environment.

A   fibrocyte - or other collagen producing cell - showing passages for extrusion of collagen pre-forms (a)

B   collagen progression from chains to fibre

   1   α chain - every 3rd AA is glycine preceded by proline and followed in most cases by hydroxyproline .87nm /cycle

   2   procollagen - triple helix - made up of 3 α chains twisted in a 10.4nm turn

   3   tropocollagen - collagen molecule consists of 3 α chains 300nm X 1.5nm - assembled ec.

   4   collagen fibril is composed of staggered X-linked tropocollagen chains which have a gap b/n them - causing them to appear banded

   5   collagen fibre

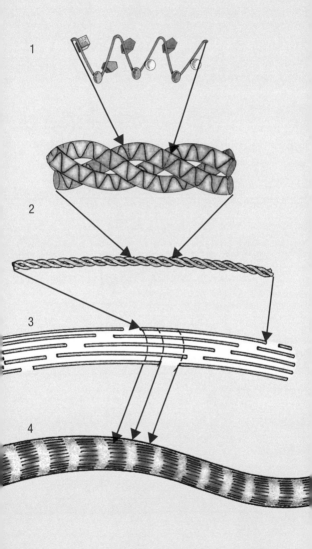

1

2

3

4

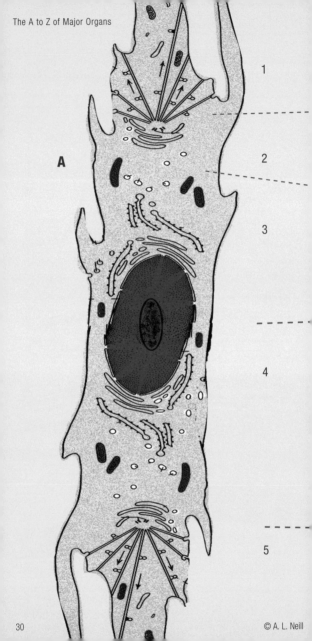

A

1

2

3

4

5

© A. L. Neill

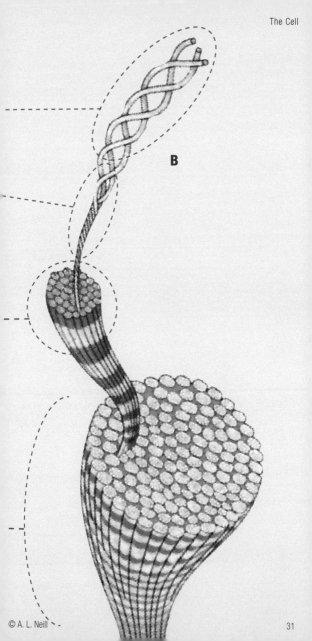

B

COLLAGEN TYPE	FIBRILLAR TYPE	DISTRIBUTION
I	large banded	throughout the body greatest tensile strength in tendons
II	small banded	in CT stroma bone, cartilage & gels of the eye
III	small banded	throughout the body as a meshwork around parenchyma, in LP
IV	sheet-like, meshwork	BM, lens
V	thin fibrillar	muscle
VI	thin fibrils	throughout ec & ic
VII	small fibrillar	anchoring fibres of the BM
VIII	hexagonal lattice	cornea
IX	fibril	cartilage
X	short chains	developing cartilage
XI	fibril	cartilage

MAIN SYNTHESIZING CELL TYPE(S)	OTHER
fibrocyte	main type in the body bone, m & tendons
chondrocyte osteocyte	
fibrocyte ito cells of the liver	main form of stroma AKA reticulin
epithelial cells endothelial cells	
smooth & skeletal m cells	
fibrocytes	
epithelial cells endothelial cells	
epithelial cells	
chondrocytes	
chondrocytes	
chondrocytes	

Elastin

Elastin fibres, as occurs in the other 3 fibrillar extracellular matrix components, are assembled & maintained extracellularly, after preliminary synthesis w/n the cell. These fibres are a combination of 2 components fibrillin filaments & elastin fibres. The fibres are bound together with glycoprotein cross-bridges in such a way that they are coiled in the relaxed state. When stretched they become linear w/o breakage of the cross-bridges and then reform as another coiled shape. With age there is less recoil.

1   fibroblast or smooth muscle cell
2   elastin protein
      p   extruded from the cell as pro-elastin
      t   tropo-elastin formed ec
3   fibrillin filaments extruded from the cell
4   glycoprotein extruded from the cell
5   all 3 fibrils form the immature elastin fibre
6   assembled fibres attract ec material to form mature elastin fibres

7   immature elastin fibres
8   mature elastin fibrous coil
9   stretched elastin meshwork
10 re-coiled - new shape

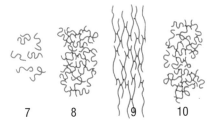

7   8   9   10

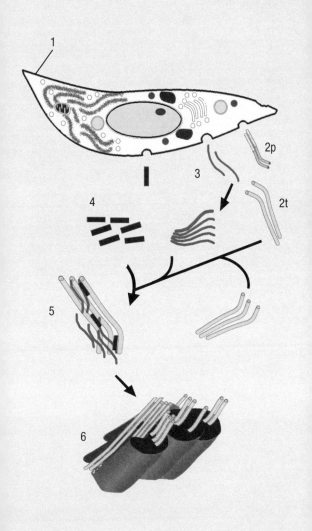

1

2p

3

2t

4

5

6

Golgi Apparatus

Schema

The Golgi apparatus consists of a number of large flattened vesicular discs which interconnect in a network - the Golgi Network - GN. There are several subsections to this network, as the protein after synthesis undergoes further modification before it is complete.

1   rER - closely connected to the Golgi - also connected to sER part of the intracellular vesicular network

2   vesicles with newly synthesised protein - budd off and move through the GN

3   cis-GN - site of phosphorylation of the new protein (adding PO_4^{3-})

4   budding protein moving to the next stage

5   medial-GN - for glycosylation of protein (adding sugars)

6   trans-GN - for transport of the proteins to...

      intracellular site of action

      secretion

      storage

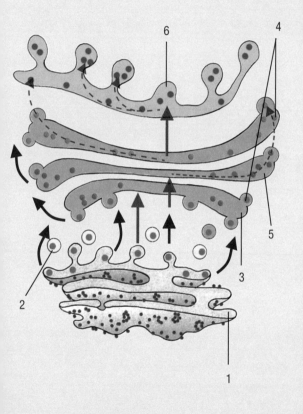

Lysosomes

Schema
biogenesis

Lysosomes are derived from endosomes and are the major source of intracellular substance disposal, recycling, and waste elimination. These organelles may inject digestive enzymes directly into the extracellular space, to pre-digest materials and facilitate phagocytosis. In order to maintain an internal environment favourable for bio-destruction & prevent substance diffusion, their mem is highly glycosylated, and crowded with specific proteins, limiting its lipid component, and permeability. The lysosomal membrane also contains extensive H^+ pumps, and maintains an internal acid environment, which combined with a large number of internal and membrane bound enzymes, acts to rapidly denature and deactivate cytoplasmic materials.

1   GA + ER
2   vesicle with proteins - undergoing exocytosis
3   specific lysosomal proteins
4   protective protein coating - internally & externally changing the nature of the lipid membrane
5   endosomes - containing protein insertions and generating an internal acid environment

>   e = early
>   L = late

6   early lysosome - developing a specific mem & int. environment
7   H^+ pumps = proton pump
8   polysaccharide pumps attached to glycosidases
9   lipid pumps attached to lipidases
10 protein pumps attached to proteases
11 nucleaic acids attached to nucleases
12 CM
13 lysosomal mem - internally coated with sugars & filled with proteins insertions & pumps

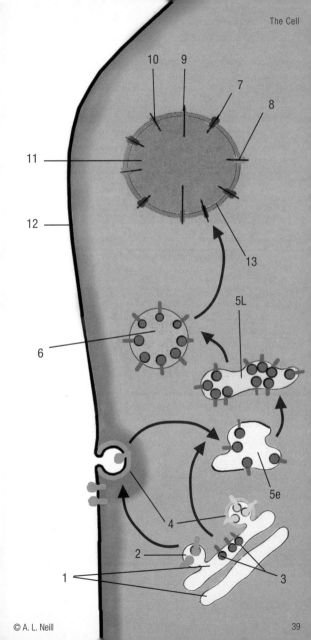

Lysosomes

Schema

functions

Lysosomes are the major source of intracellular substance disposal, recycling, and waste elimination. They destroy/digest organelles and internal waste proteins via *autophagy*, bacteria & large foreign bodies via *phagocytosis*, and small proteins via **endocytosis** releasing the components for re-use if possible, extruding them from the cell if toxic or forming locked vesicles which remain w/n the cell & accumulate with age.

1 bacteria - undergoing phagocytosis
    i = phagosome
    ii = fusion with the lysosomal mem
2 proteins - undergoing endocytosis
    i = vesicle
    ii = endosome
    iii = late - modified endosome
3 ER - moving to older damaged organelle
    i = autophagosome
    ii = autophagolysosome - fusion with the lysosome
4 lysosome
5 damaged mitochondria
6 storage vesicle - filled with old protein - e.g. lipofuscin

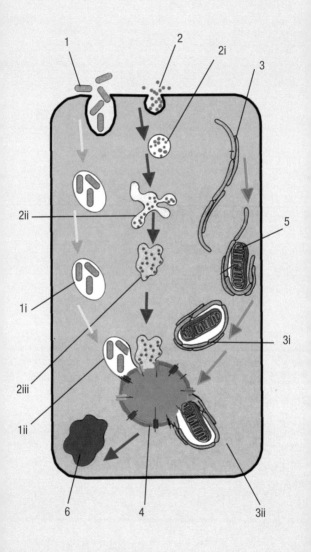

Mitochondria (mito)
Energy Production

Schema

mitochondrial structure
E generation chain

Mito generate the E of the cell by forming water (H_2O) from H^+ & O^{2-} (derived from the B) and capturing the E released from that reaction. They store the E as ATP, using membranous enzyme & ion pumps. They move the E in and out of the mito via transmembranous protein pumps. The inner & outer mems function independently, with different permeabilities & surface charges. Mito have their own distinct DNA, ribosomes, ion and substrate stores and regulate their own activity, even initiating apoptosis, w/o direct nuclear input. It is thought they evolved from invading intracellular bacteria.

1   inner mitochondrial mem
2   intermembranous space
3   outer mitochondrial mem
4   cristae derived from the inner mem containing enzymes in partic. ATP-ase for E release

     p = elementary particles with ATP synthetase complex - for E creation

5   matrix
6   matrix granules - containing stores of cations, in particular Ca^{2+}
7   mem protein pumps to transfer H^+ into the mito for oxidative phosphorylation and ATP generation
8   ATP synthase complex
9   ADP / ATP pump

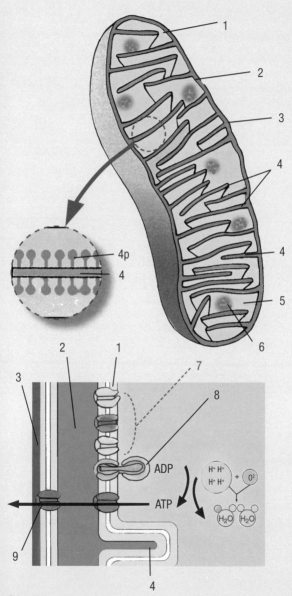

ADP

ATP

$H^+ H^+$
$H^+ H^+$ + O^2

H_2O H_2O

© A. L. Neill

Nucleus

Schema
Nucleus overview
Nuclear membrane in HP
Nuclear pore in HP

The nucleus is the brain of the cell - and if resting w/n the nucleus is a store of "resting" quiescent chromatin, the nucleoli.

Changes in the activity of the cell change the number of nucleoli and nuclear pores. More activity increases the pores and decreases the nucleoli as the DNA disperses.

The nucleus has a double membrane which communicates directly with the ER and Golgi membrane networks but to directly communicate with the cytoplasm, proteins and other material pass through the nuclear pores which cross the perinuclear space through a number of protein baskets.

1   nuclear chromatin + nucleolus
2   rER - ER + ribosomes
3   inner (i) & outer (o) mem of nuclear envelope
4   nuclear pore - communicating with the cytoplasm
5   nuclear lamina - similar to the tus directly under the CM
6   cytoplasm
7   communication b/n ER and nuclear mem
8   transient protein – moving out to the cytoplasm
9   rings & filaments of the nuclear pore
    c = cytoplasmic ring
    cf = cytoplasmic filament
    f = nuclear filament
    l = luminal ring
    n = nuclear ring
    t = terminal ring

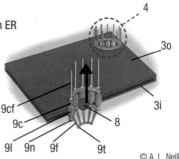

© A. L. Neill

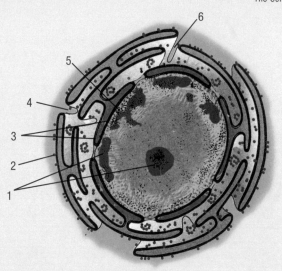

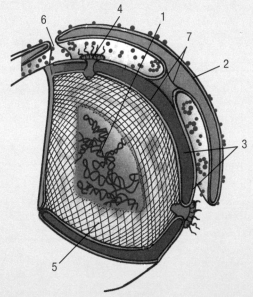

Ribosomes
Protein Synthesis

Schema

Ribosomes exist for the main purpose of synthesizing proteins for the cell. The 2 ribosomal subunits assemble around a ribbon of mRNA which represents a protein recipe (translated from the nucleus). The mRNA - may emerge through the ER or Golgi apparatus membranes, or present in the cytoplasm. Once bound onto this ribbon of RNA - the ribosome will step by step move along its length assembling a protein as it does so. When a specific codon is reached the protein will be cleaved - and the ribosome will break apart - ready to re-assemble and begin making another protein. If the protein is assembled on the ER it will be released inside this bilayered membrane and be transported to its site of action. Either way the main steps are the same. The protein builds up from a growing chain of AAs starting on the A site, joining the chain on the P site then moving along the E site to allow another AA to join the A site.

1　growing polypeptide - string of AAs which will become a protein
2　ribosomal subunits L = large s = small
3　RNA
   　　m = messenger - mRNA
   　　r = ribosomal - rRNA
   　　t = transfer - tRNA
4　amino acid = AA
5　a single ribonucleic acid = RNA
   　　c = codon = collection of 3 RNA's in a row which code for a particular AA or action for the ribosome
6　ribosome receptor
7　membrane pore
8　rER = ribosomes bound onto the surface of ER
9　signal codon sequence
10　cleaved protein inside the ER membrane

a = A site　　　**e** = E site　　　**p** = P site

　　　　　　　　　　　　　　　　　　　　© A. L. Neill

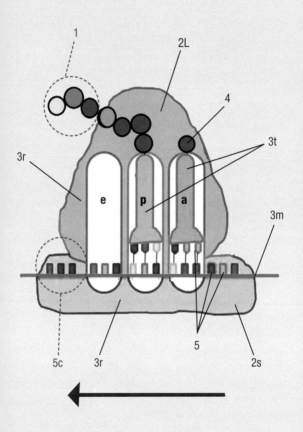

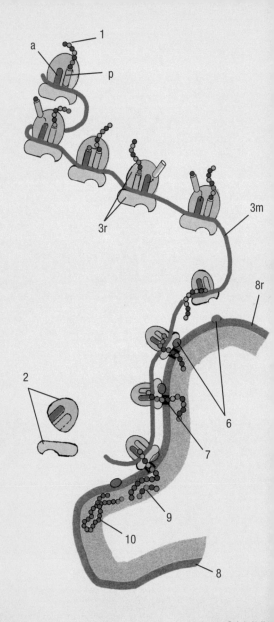

a

1

p

3r

3m

8r

2

6

7

9

10

8

48

© A. L. Neill

Vesicles
Types

Vesicles are membrane enclosed bubbles w/n a cell. Hence most organelles in the cell are forms of vesicles. Not the nucleolus is not a vesicle. Artificial nanoparticles are designed to produce bodies which will go into the cells.

1	cargo vesicles	vesicles generated by surface cell receptors - which bind and then enclose specific proteins
2	endosomes	pre-lysosomes
3	ER	vesicular plates involved in rapid intracellular transport
4	Golgi apparatus	vesicular plates involved in efficiently synthesizing proteins & exporting them
5	lysosomes	suicide vesicle
6	matrix vesicle	ec vesicle involved in biomineralization of the matrix as in bone & cartilage
7	microbody	see peroxisome
8	mitochondria	2X membranous vesicles which generates E aerobically for the cell - and initiates apoptosis
9	multivesicular vesicles	a vesicle containing other vesicles - e.g. phagolysosome
10	nuclei	2X membranous vesicle which houses the main control of the cell
11	peroxisomes	uni-membranous - i.e. not a lipid bliayer vesicle involved in fatty chain catabolism
12	pinocytic vesicles	small vesicles containing small molecules of liquid
13	phagosomes	vesicles containing material enveloped by the cell for deactivation &/or destruction
14	secretory vesicles	capsule to transport product out of the cell - e.g. Hs
15	storage vesicles	membrane-bound sacks of storage material e.g. fat
16	synaptic vesicles	specific secretory vesicle of the NS - to transport
17	transport vesicles	used to move particle or FB around; in or out of the cell may be generated by other organelles
18	vacuole	water containing vesicle

Cell – processes
Apoptosis / Necrosis

Schema

Part of the normal cell processes include a controlled death of the cell w/o initiating the inflammatory process. This begins with activation of the "internalized death" mediated by cytochrome C release from the mito.

Stimulation for *apoptotic processes* to begin may come externally via the "death receptor" - activated by circulating lymphokines such as the TNF family, free radicals, UV rays, Hs and other *death factors*; or internally by anti-metabolites, anti-tumour factors. These vie with *survival factors* such as growth Hs, extracellular matrix molecules, & Zn, to determine if this process actually starts but once initiated the process like necrosis is irreversible.

	Apoptosis - A	Necrosis - N
1	Initiation of death process cytochrome C release from mito ↓ cell volume	Damage to the CM ↑ cell volume
2	DNA fragmentation	CM breakdown
3	CM blebbing w/o exposure	Escape of organelles Complete breakdown of cell structure
4	Formation of opsonised membrane enclosed bodies of groups of organelles - apoptotic bodies primed with ligands to facilitate phagocytosis	Disintegration and activation of the inflammatory process

A

N

1

2

3

4

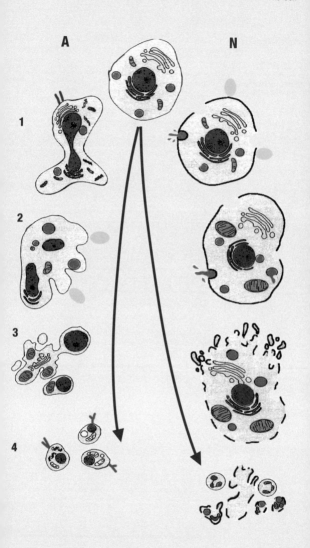

Cell – processes
Migration

Schema

In any inflammatory or immune process, cells are induced to migrate to the affected area. These cells may be neutrophils or monocytes. In the healing process, epithelial cells and fibroblasts migrate to fill the deficit. There is a difference b/n the 2 cell types - connective and epithelial. Only the neutrophil process is illustrated.

	Neutrophils - CT cell type	Epithelial cell type
A	surface adhesion molecules interact with the altered endothelium	cell to cell contact is lost in a defect
B	stick to the endothelium - and roll rather than flow in the BV	↑ cell volume ↓ specializations ↑ cell to flatten & spread out
C	further adherence causes ↑ cell to cell interaction and ↑ adherence molecules of the neutrophil to form, specific to the immune response	cells undergo mitosis, lay down BM
D	endothelial cells are opened at the site of the reaction by resident mast cells & a neutrophil pseudopod is extended through this gap	cells move along the new BM
E	neutrophil - now PMN migrates in the T towards the site of injury	cell to cell contact is re-established, migration is stopped and epithelium reforms in original form

1	neutrophil	6	histamine ± heparin to separate endothelial cells
2	endothelial lining	7	mast cell
3	BM	8	pseudopod
4	integrin + integrin receptor complex	9	PMN
5	immune responsive adherent surface molecules	10	chemotactic stimulants

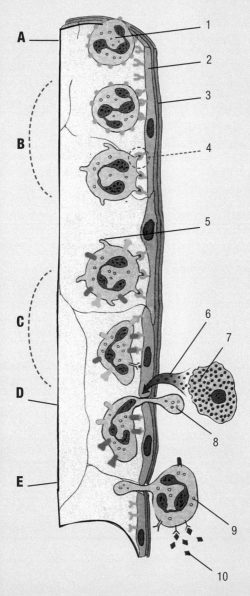

A

1

2

3

B

4

5

C

6

7

D

8

E

9

10

Cell replication
Mitosis - Meiosis

Schema

Most cells divide asexually - mitosis (M) and have an exact replication of the original cell's DNA. These daughter cells have 2 sets of chromosomes. They are diploid (2n).

Germ cells (ovum, spermatocyte) need to halve their chromosomes. To divide they must first recombine and form a new genome then repeat the process w/o DNA duplication to reduce their new genome and become haploid (n)- having only one of each chromosome so that they may then combine in fertilization and form a new individual with a different genome - meiosis (F), each germ cell contributing half of the total DNA of the new zygote, which is now diploid (2n) but different from either original germ cell.

1   **first polar body**
2   **second polar body**
3   **spermatozoa**
4   **ovum**

	MITOSIS
PROPHASE A	chromatin is duplicated (2n) & aligns itself into parallel sister chromosomes
	centrioles replicate to form 2 microtubule centres & the mitotic spindle which attaches to the chromosomes after the NM breakdown
METAPHASE B	chromosomes move along the microtubules to the centre of the cell
ANAPHASE C	chromosomes move to the opposite poles of the spindle & the cell elongates
TELOPHASE D	new NMs form - chromatin detaches from the spindle
CYTOKINESIS E	new CMs form via actin & myosin filaments in the cell and there are 2 identical daughter cells (2n)
PROPHASE A2 METAPHASE B2 ANAPHASE C2 TELOPHASE D2 CYTOKINESIS E2	

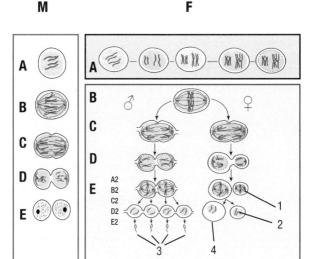

M

F

A

B

C

D

E

MEIOSIS - reduction division

chromatin is duplicated and aligns itself into parallel sister chromosomes - and then the chromatin is swapped from 1 gene to another changing the make up of each chromosome otherwise the same as for mitosis

chromosomes move along the microtubules to the centre of the cell

chromosomes move to the opposite poles of the spindle & the cell elongates

new NMs form - chromatin detaches from the spindle

new CMs form but 1 new cell is produced and 1 polar body (1) in the female (2n) 2 new cells in the male (2n)

The process is repeated w/o duplication to return reduce the cells to haploid so they can become full germ cells.

THE OVUM (n) in the female and the second polar body (2)

4 SPERMATOZOA (n) in the male

Cell – processes
Endocytosis - selective

Schema

Most cells are involved in ingesting substances selectively. These materials (1) may alter cell activities: causing further specialization; upgrading or downgrading protein production etc. and are often mediated by a specific CM receptor (2).

1   cargo substance - e.g. neurotransmitter or H
      e = extracellular
      i = intracellular
2   receptor
3   adaptin molecule
4   cargo complex - 1 + 2 + 3 - allowing endocytosis
5   protective proteins - to prevent autodigesion of the vesicle
6   coated pit
7   coated vesicle
8   vesicle
9   vesicle combined at effector site
10   further modification of cargo substance
      OR
11   vesicle breakdown and release of cargo substance

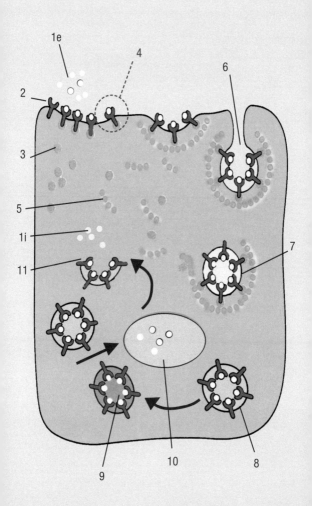

Cell – processes
Exocytosis

Schema

Cells are both involved in producing materials primarily for external use. They do this via exocytosis.

This may be

constitutional **I**

where the exports are produced and exported w/o storage, as in the production of monomers for extracellular fibrils as with fibrocytes

or

regulated **II**

where the exports are produced and stored and rely on a trigger for release, as with the production of enzymes or Hs, as with glandular cells.

1   ER + ribosomes (rER)
2   Golgi apparatus
    t = transitional vesicles
3   storage vesicles
4   trigger complex
    L = either neuronal or hormonal trigger = ligand
    r = receptor - to receive trigger and activate release
5   Ca^{++} channel to mediate release
6   endosome - transport vesicle
7   protein - release product

I II

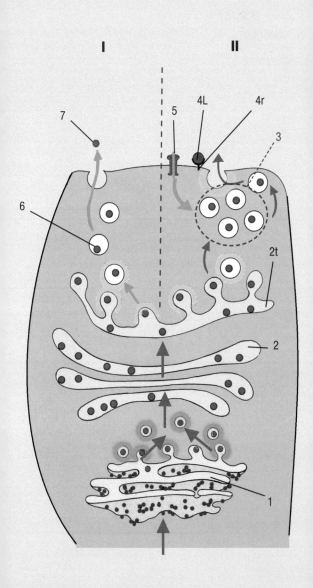

Cell – processes
Phagocytosis

Schema
Antigenic (I)
Non-antigenic (II)

Phagocytosis occurs either via activated particles which have been coated with circulating Abs and connect to CM surface Ags as in most bacteria (I) or in a non-specific non-antigenic way as with most foreign particles (II).

1   bacterium particle
2   circulating Abs
3   coated bacterium
4   Fc receptor - specific CM receptor for the attached Ab
5   terminal web - actin filaments
6   phagosome
7   lysosome
8   phagolysosome - digesting the ingested particle
9   foreign body - non-antigenic
10 non-specific CM receptors

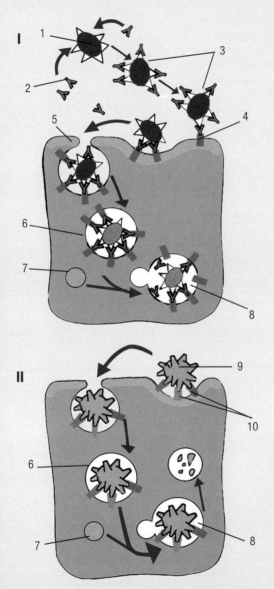

Epithelial cells
Overview

Micro Schema

Simple epithelium is nearly always polarized - i.e. there is a distinctive base and apex to the cells. The cells adhere to a BM & stick to each other via specialized adherent structures; the apex often has devices to increase the CM surface area, to facilitate absorption secretion or movement of substances near these cells.

A apical region

B basal region

L lateral region

1 microvilli (mv) f = filaments in the mv
2 terminal web
3 ZO
4 ZA
5 desmosome joining 2 CMs -
    h = hemi-desmosomes joining CM to the BM
      3 + 4 + 5 = adherence complex
6 gap junction
7 filaments and fibrils
8 focal adhesions
9 collagen anchoring filaments
10 BM

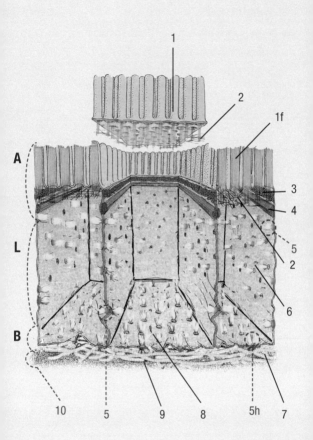

Epithelial cells – specializations
Focal Adhesions

Micro Schema

These structures are used to connect 2 epithelial cells together, at a single point – rather than a "zone" along the CM.

They stick the CMs of 2 cells together or connect the CM to the BM; they are smaller, weaker and more transient than desmosomes or hemidesmosomes.

1 CM
2 adherent fibrils
    i = extracellular
    ii = transmembranous
3 adherent protein plaque
    i = cytoplasmic
       2 + 3 = adherent complex
4 actin filaments
5 BM
6 fibronectin = BM fibrils (collagen based fibrils)

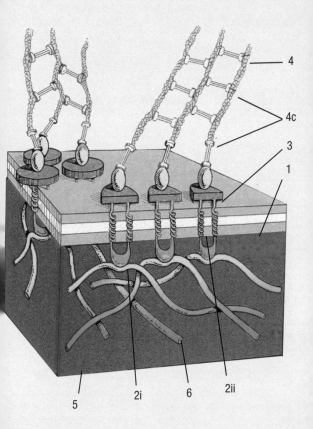

4

4c

3

1

2i

6

2ii

5

Epithelial cells – specializations
Gap Junctions

Micro Schema

LP

HP

These structures are used to communicate b/n 2 epithelial cells at a single point in the CM. Generally in the apical region these junctions may be seen at other points in the cell. The channels composed of 6 transmembranous protein subunits may be controlled by Ca^{2+} and may be under ionic, neural, hormonal or other influences.

1   CM

2   transmembranous proteins

       i = subunits (6 per gap)

3   allows the passage of specific molecules and intercellular communication when open (3o) which is stopped when closed (3c).

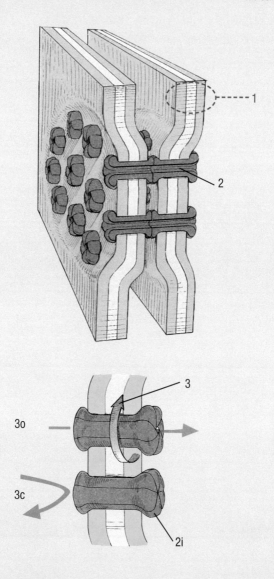

Epithelial cells – specializations
Hemidesmosomes

Micro Schema

These structures are used to connect the base CM of epithelial cells with the BM, at specific points. Similar to Desmosomes, transmembranous proteins (integrin) (2) project extracellularly and lodge in the BM. The BM contributes with collagen XVII (5f) fibrils projecting into the CM and collagen VII reticular fibrils (6) anchors the epithelia to the CT underneath.

1 CM
2 adherent fibrils
3 adherent protein plaque
4 actin filaments
5 BM
     f = anchoring filaments (collagen)
6 reticular fibrils
7 collagen (III) fibres
8 mitochondrium

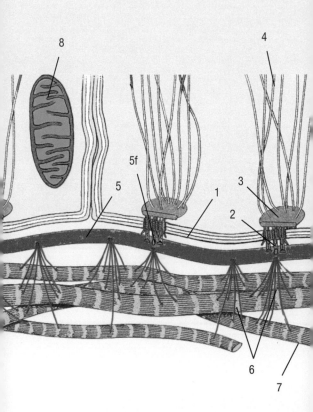

Epithelial cells – specializations
Macula Adherens = Desmosomes

Micro Schema

LP

HP

These structures are used to connect 2 epithelial cells together at a single "patch" – rather than a "zone" along the CM. They stick the CMs of 2 cells together or as Hemidesmosomes connect the CM to the BM.

1   CM
2   adherent fibrils
      i = extracellular
      ii = transmembranous
      iii = cytoplasmic
3   adherent protein plaque
      2 + 3 = adherent complex
4   actin filaments

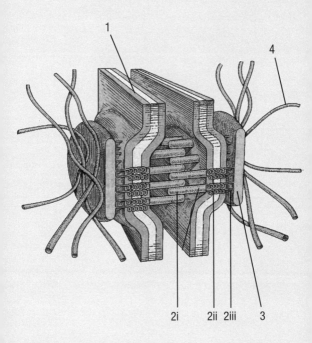

1

4

2i   2ii 2iii   3

Epithelial cells – specializations
Zonula Adherans (ZA)

Micro Schema

This structure connects 2 cells together. As a "zone" the structure extends along the whole length of the connecting CM in the apical region of the epithelial cell and is part of the junctional complex (Jc).

It is used as a device to prevent material from moving from one side of the simple epithelium to the other w/o passing through the cells - to keep the cells together.

The strength of this barrier may be altered via channels controlled by Ca^{2+} ions, unlike the ZO.

1   cell membrane = CM
2   Calcium channels
3   adherans bridge - activated by the Ca^{2+} through the channels
4   transmembrane proteins - integrin
5   cytoplasmic adherent proteins

      3 + 4 + 5 = adherence complex

6   actin filaments - c = connecting bridges - α actinin

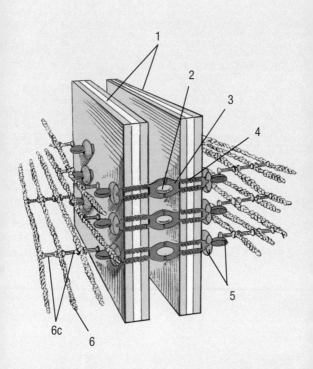

Epithelial cells – specializations
Zonula Occludens (ZO)

Micro Schema

LP

HP

This structure connects 2 cells together. As a "zone" the structure extends along the whole length of the connecting CM in the apical region of the epithelial cell & is part of the junctional complex (Jc).

It is used as a device to prevent material from moving from one side of the simple epithelium to the other w/o passing through the cells. It is a stronger & less flexible barrier than the ZA.

1   cell membrane = CM
2   occludin fibrils
  i = extracellular
  ii = transmembranous
  iii = cytoplasmic
3   occludin proteins
  2 + 3 = occluden complex
4   actin filaments

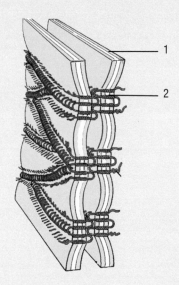

1

2

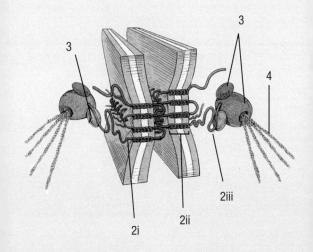

3

3

3

4

2i

2ii

2iii

Epithelial cells – associated structures
Basement Membrane (BM)

Micro Schema

Epithelial cells are arranged in rows, joined to each other via special adhesion structures. Their base sits on a mucopolysaccharide structure 0.05mm thick. The BM attaches them to the underlying CT. This multilayered structure stains poorly with routine H&E. Specific stains such as PAS - to stain the sugars or silver stains to show the reticular fibres will demonstrate its presence much better. Regions have more or less BM adhesion devices depending upon the stresses of the overlying epithelium, e.g. the skin is very tightly bound whereas the lining of the DT is not.

1   cytoplasm

2   CM

3   lamina lucida

4   lamina densa - may have downward projections, associated with the collagen reticular fibres of... 5 (partic in the skin)

5   fibroreticular lamina

6   CT - connected to the BM

7   anchoring fibres (type IV collagen) - assoc with hemidesmosomes providing a link from the epi cell → BM → CT

8   elastic fibres & fibrillin microfilaments

9   collagen - reticular (type III collagen - smaller & more coiled) & normal fibres in the CT

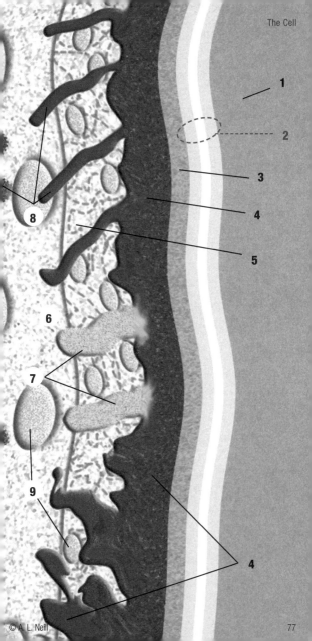

1

2

3

4

5

6

7

8

9

4

Epithelial cells
Cilia

Micro Schema

LP - coronal with cross-sections

Epithelial cells may have devices to assist in the movements of substances. These long cytoplasmic extensions are cilia and they move independently, propelled by the microtubules found in their basal portions = basal bodies. They are highly organized with microtubular doublets and triplets connected via cytoplasmic proteins which in the stem break and reform, but which are rigid in the basal body (bb) of the cilium.

1   central sheath

2   central microtubules

3   microtubular bundle - doublet in stem and triplet in the base

> i - 1st ring made up of tubulin subunits
>
> ii - 2nd ring similar structure
>
> iii - 3rd ring - dynein arms in the stem - tubilin ring in the base

4   connecting link to join microtubular ring groups - forms and reforms with movement

5   spoke protein joining the rings to the central sheath in the cilial stem

6   actin filaments of the terminal web support the bb

7   CM

8   cytoplasm - extends up the cilial stem

9   bb

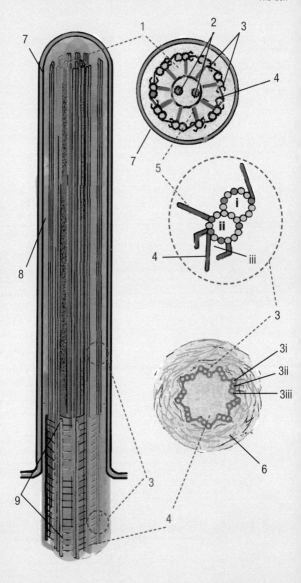

Epithelial cells –
Microvilli

Micro Schema

Epithelial cells often have devices to assist in the absorption of substrates - the simplest are the microvilli (mv) additional structured folds of the CM. Actin filaments insert into these folds embedding in the apical proteins and are joined together with protein cross-bridges. The filaments insert basally into the terminal web of actin filaments - underneath which lie myosin filaments.

1 villin - apical protein
2 protein cross-links = fimbrin / fascin & others
3 actin filaments
4 myosin - cross-links
5 cytoplasm
6 CMs
7 terminal web
8 myosin filaments - intermediate
9 stabilizing fibrils

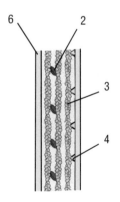

© A. L. Neill

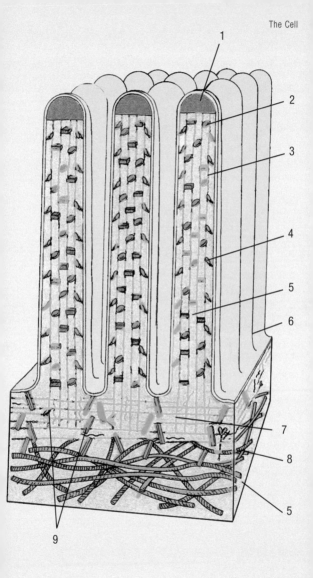

1

2

3

4

5

6

7

8

5

9

Epithelial cells –
Stereocilia / Stereovilli

Micro Schema

Epithelial cells often have devices to assist in the transport of substances along a canal or tubule as in the respiratory tract. As with the mv - the stereovilli are cytoplasmic projections covered in the CM with actin filaments inserted. Cytoplasmic cross-bridges with embedded stabilizing proteins help to prevent breakages in these much longer projections (>100). They are more motile than mvs and generally do not have an absorptive function. They resemble cilia but are not as structured - there are no microtubules; the basal bodies are not as organized but are a mass of actin cross-bridges inserted in the thickened terminal web. As with cilia there are no apical proteins.

1 apex cytoplasm
2 protein cross-links = fimbrin / erzin & others
3 actin filaments
4 terminal web
5 cytoplasm b = bridges
6 CM
7 stabilizing fibrils

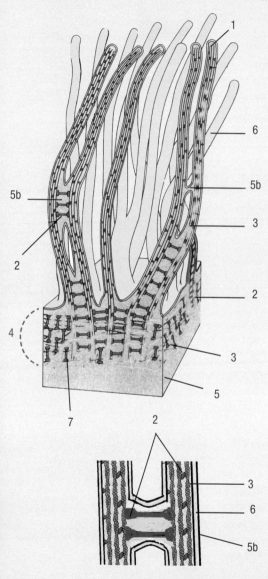

Epithelial cells –
Glands

Schema

Epithelial cells which secrete materials in order to influence the actions of other cells are **glands**. They may be single cells placed amongst other epithelial cells - **unicellular** - or as clusters of secreting cells - multicellular.

A **Endocrine** glands secrete **hormones** (H) directly into the BS. The target cells are separated from the gland.

B **Exocrine** gland secretions open directly onto a surface, or into a duct. The cells are polarized with a base (6) & luminal (5) surface. Exocrine secretions are of 3 major types.

   i *Apocrine* - cytoplasm-coated vesicles are released from the cell's apex

   ii *Merocrine* - direct material release from the apex via exocytosis

   iii *Holocrine* - apoptosis & vesicle release occur together after a large amount of secretory product has accumulated - discharging cell debris & substance into the duct

C **Paracrine** gland secretions are only locally effective. The material diffuses into the immediate vicinity, affecting adjacent cells &/or subjacent CT.

1 BV - often fenestrated capillaries to facilitate the H molecules passing into the lumen

2 BM - all epithelial cells sit on a BM

3 H in vesicles

4 H released into the extracellular space - moving to the BS

5 lumen of duct / the cells' apex

6 base of cell

7 exocytosis

8 cytoplasm coated vesicles of secretory material

9 apoptosis with release of stored secretions

10 secretory material

11 receptors - adjacent cell / in subjacent CT

12 CT cells

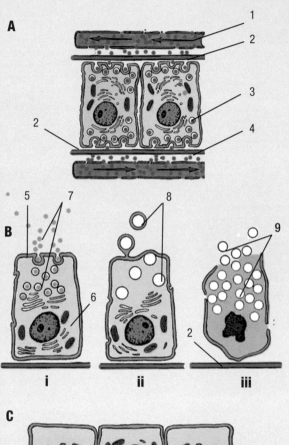

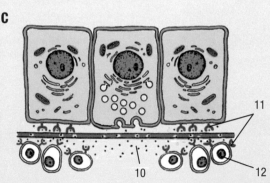

Epithelial cells
Glands - Exocrine

Schema

Exocrine glands may be simple (A) or compound (B). The tubular cells may alter the secretion by concentrating it - e.g. the salivary & sweat glands or they may merely act as tubes to transport the secretions, which enter along their lengths as in sebaceous glands.

1. simple acinar - urethra
2. branched acinar - stomach
3. compound acinar - pancreas
4. simple branched tubular - stomach
5. simple coiled tubular - sweat
6. compound tubuloacinar - submandibular salivary
7. compound tubular - duodenum
8. simple tubular - large intestine

A   **B**

1

2

4

3

5

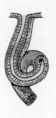

6

8

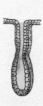

7

© A. L. Neill

Epithelial cells
Types

Schema

The epithelium always sits upon a BM. If simple it is single layered of varying morphologies, otherwise it is stratified as in the skin & urogenital tract.

1	simple squamous	alveolar vascular (endothelium)	barrier exchange
2	simple cuboidal	germinal glandular tubular	absorption conduit secretion
3	simple columnar	DT lining	absorption secretion
4	pseudostratified	respiratory tract lining	filter modifier secretion
5	stratified squamous	skin mucous membranes	barrier secretion
6	transitional	urogenital linings (urothelium)	barrier conduit

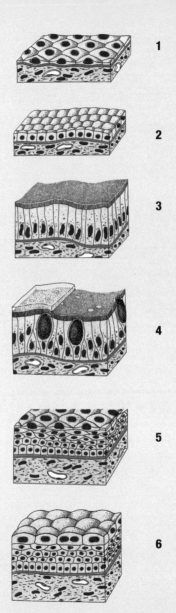

1

2

3

4

5

6

ANATOMICAL POSITION & PLANES

This is the anatomical position.

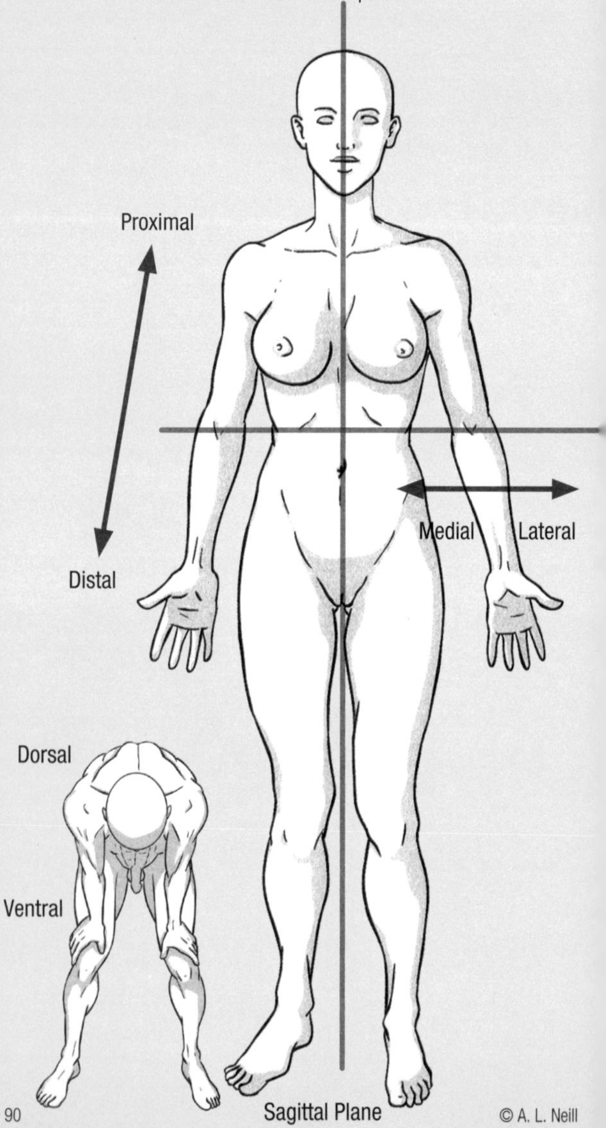

Proximal

Distal

Medial

Lateral

Dorsal

Ventral

Sagittal Plane

90 © A. L. Neill

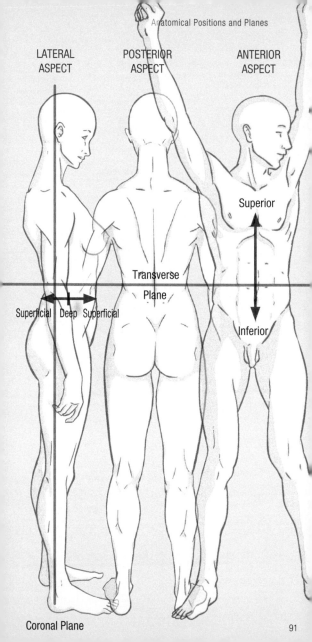

LATERAL
ASPECT

POSTERIOR
ASPECT

ANTERIOR
ASPECT

Superior

Transverse
Plane

Inferior

Superficial   Deep   Superficial

Coronal Plane

91

POSITION OF ORGANS ON THE BODY

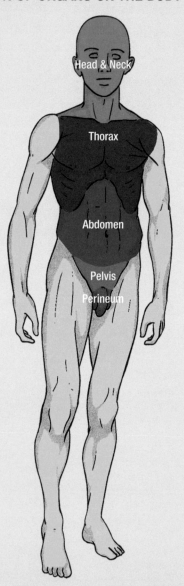

Head & Neck

Thorax

Abdomen

Pelvis

Perineum

© A. L. Neill

SITES OF REFERRED ORGAN PAIN

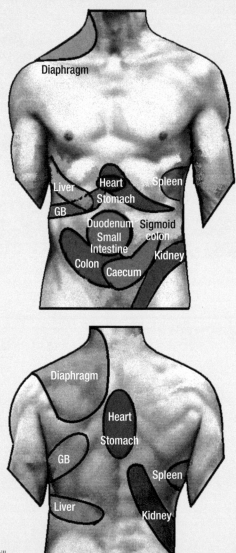

Adrenal gland

Macroscopic view
Anterior view - in situ

The adrenal gland is superior to the kidney - hence its name. It has 2 distinct functions - the medulla which acts as a glandular form of the sympathetic ANS, amplifying the effects of sympathetic stimulation e.g. in the Fight or Flight syndrome and the cortex strongly involved in the control of steroid release & cortisol levels. The gland also interacts with the parasympathetic enteric ganglia.

1   L Vagal trunk wrapped around the terminal part of the oesophagus
2   R Vagus N
3   renal ganglia L & R
4   coeliac ganglia L & R
5   intermesenteric plexus
6   sympathetic trunk L & R
7   inferior mesenteric ganglion & Ns wrapped around the inf mesenteric a
8   superior mesenteric ganglion & Ns wrapped around the sup. mesenteric a
9   coeliac trunk
10 adrenal gland L & R
11 greater splanchnic N
12 lesser splanchnic N
13 thoracic sympathetic chain

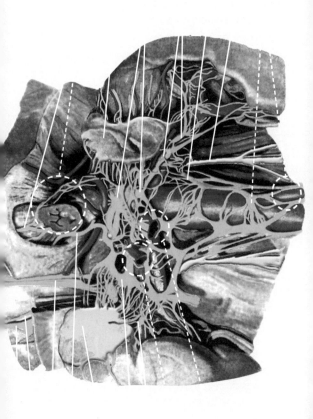

1

10L

4L

3L

5

6L

7

13
12
11
2

10R

4R

3R

9

8

Adrenal gland

A

Histology

*Transverse section LP H&E -
showing most of the basic structures
HP - sections to show various
specialized regions*

The adrenal gland is an encapsulated gland
(A) divided into the cortex (B), which is
involved in the corticosteroid balance of the
body & the medulla (C), which is part of the
sympathetic NS.

Bi

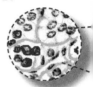

A   capsule

B   Cortex - 3 zones based on the
cellular arrangement

    i   zona glomerulosa

    ii   zone fasciculata

    iii zona reticularis

Bii

C   Medulla

Biii

1   Capsule and CT septum
2   arteriole
3   unmyelinated Ns
4   cells of the zona glomerulosa
5   sinusoids - present in all 3 zones
6   cells of the zona reticularis
7   pigmented cells in the 6
8   sympathetic ganglion cells
9   medullary veins

C

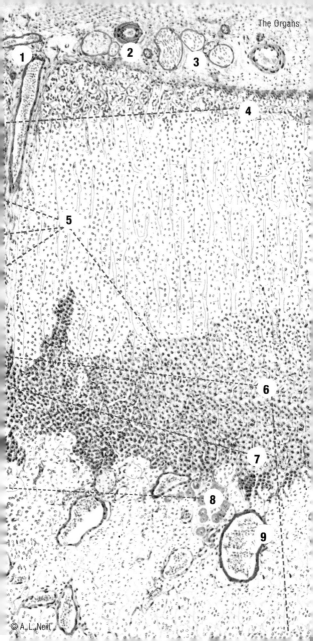

The Organs

© A. L. Neill

Adrenal gland

Schema

The adrenal has several zones

A Capsule

B Cortex - 3 zones based on the cellular arrangement

      i   zona glomerulosa

      ii zone fasciculata

      iii zona reticularis

C Medulla

The BS is extensive and the capillaries sinusoids to facilitate passage of the Hs synthesized by this gland. These are stimulated by N synapse in the medulla and stimulating Hs of the pituitary axis in the cortex regions.

1   secrete mineralocorticoids

2   secrete glucocorticoids

3   secrete gonadocorticoids

4   secrete adrenalin - note synapse with the preganglionic sympathetic N - these cells act as postganglionic Ns

5   secrete noradrenalin

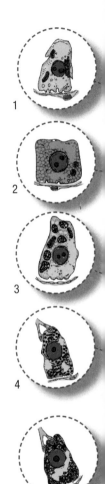

© A. L. Neill

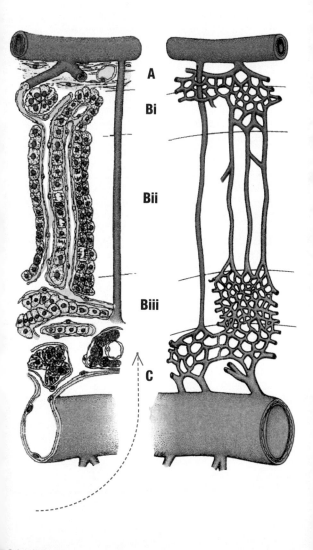

A

Bi

Bii

Biii

C

Appendix

Macroscopic view
Anterior - wall cut away from the caecum and the
mesentery removed
Schema of possible appendix positions

The appendix is a blind intestinal tube located in the RIF, at the ilocaecal junction. The BS comes from the mesentery which supports it and gives it mobility - allowing the organ to swing around in front of and behind the LI. This may compromise the BS and function of the organ causing an inflammatory response - appendicitis. Because of its location an inflamed appendix may affect other organs in the vicinity such as the ovary.

1   Mesentery (cut)
2   Ileum
3   straight arteries = arteriae rectae
4   arterial arcades
5   Appendicular a
6   Appendix v = appendix orifice
7   Ileocolic artery
  Brs –
    a = ant. caecal a
    c = colic a
    i = ileal a
    p = post. caecal a
8   Lymphatic follicles = Peyers' patches
9   Ascending colon
10 Caecum
11 Appendix (8-10cm) positions
    i = iliac
    p = pelvic
    r = retrocaecal - corresponds to McBirney's point 2/3
    of the line from the ASIS to the umbilicus

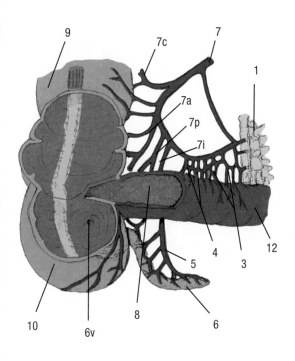

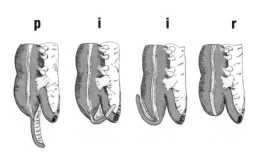

p i i r

Appendix

Histology

Transverse section LP H&E - showing most of the basic structures

The appendix is a blind intestinal tube located at the ilocaecal junction. It appears to be vestigial, but in other animals is involved in the digestion of cellulose via its stored bacteria. The mucosa has numerous lymphoid follicles & GALT.

1 peritoneal mesothelium + adipose cells
2 serosa
3 muscularis externa - consisting of 2 layers of smooth m, outer longitudinal & inner circular
4 submucosa
5 muscularis mucosa - 2 thin layers smooth m inner circular & outer longit. smooth m
6 parasympathetic ganglia of the myenteric plexus
7 intestinal glands in the mucosa
8 germinal centre of lymphoid nodule part of the GALT
9 loose lymphoid T in the LP of the mucosa
10 lining columnar epithelium - filled with goblet cells
11 lumen
12 arterioles & venules of the mucosa

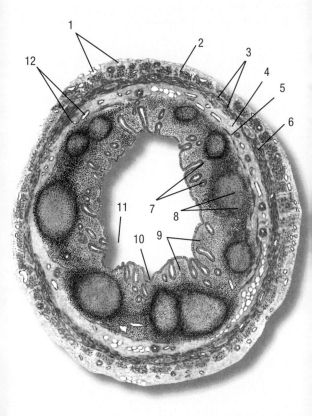

Bladder

Macroscopic view
Superior - male
Inferior - female
Internal - female - showing trigone

The bladder is a bag of multi-layered smooth muscle lined with a waterproof epithelium. It both fills and empties from the base, in the trigone, and as such any obstruction in that area will cause both filling and emptying problems. The normal bladder can contain up to 1.5 litres, which is restricted by abdominal P and may be expanded up to 3 litres if flow is obstructed.

1 median umbilical lig.
2 body
3 fundus
4 ureter
5 external muscle layer
6 urethra
7 physiological sphincter of the bladder -
     pulls the urethra post.
8 ureteric orifice
9 urethral orifice
10 sphincteric muscles - which open the ureters
11 sphincteric muscles - which open the urethra

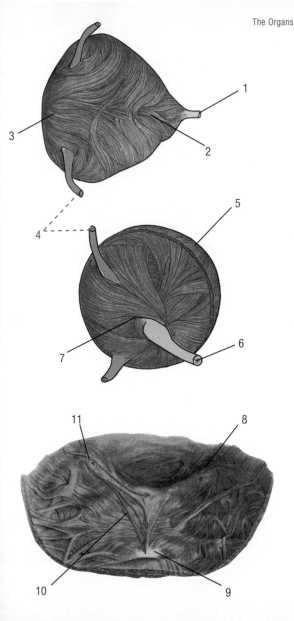

Bladder

Macroscopic view
Lateral - male - BS

The bladder is a collapsible bag which has a copious anastomotic BS
intimately related to the adjacent structures - prostate in the male -
vagina and uterus in the female.

1 int. iliac a & v
2 obliterated umbilical a
3 superior vesical a
4 fundus
5 median umbilical lig
6 vesical venous plexus
7 prostate brs from inf. vesical a & v
8 prostate
9 urethra
10 seminal vesicles
11 middle rectal v
12 ductus deferens + a
13 ureter + uteric a & v
14 inf vesical uteric a & v
15 inf. gluteal a & v

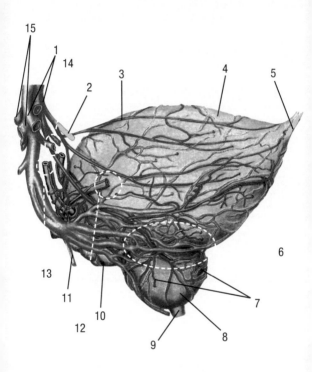

Bladder

Histology
LP - H&E showing the full depth of the bladder wall
HP - H&E showing the bladder lining and mucosa
Schema - flattened full bladder / empty bladder surface
cell changes

The bladder has an internal lining of tightly bound multilayered cuboidal epithelial cells = transitional epithelium. These cells stretch out flat when there is a volume change w/o developing gaps and so protect the underlying T from the toxic urine. This is due to the thickened apex CM and the extensive filaments in the tw, which form invaginations in the relaxed bladder and flatten when it is stretched. With each urination some of the inner cells are shed with the urine.

1 mucosal folds
2 transitional epithelium
   L luminal layer of transitional epi - note mitosis is possible throughout the layers
3 LP
4 muscularis externa, multiple bundles of smooth m
5 surface CT & CT septa
6 serosa & peritoneal mesothelium
7 veins & lymphatics of the LP
8 interplaque areas of the CM
9 plaques & invaginated plaques
10 filaments

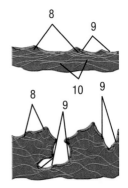

© A. L. Neill

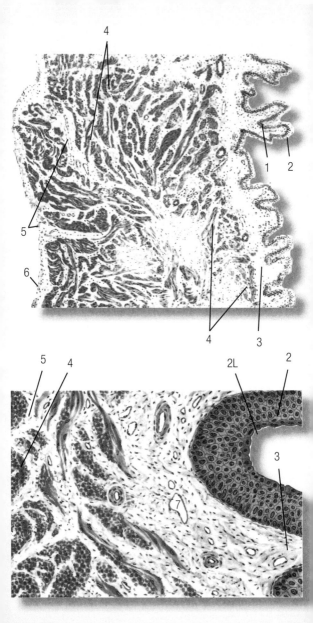

Bladder Ureter

Histology

Transverse section LP H&E - showing most of the basic structures

The ureter transports the urine from the renal pelvis to the bladder by peristalsis.

1   outer circular & inner longitudinal layers of smooth muscle
2   adipose T surrounding the ureter and supporting the BS & NS
3   arteriole
4   venule
5   surface membrane
6   transitional epithelium - multilayered expandable and waterproof
7   BM
8   lumen
9   Ns b/n the muscle layers and in the adventitia

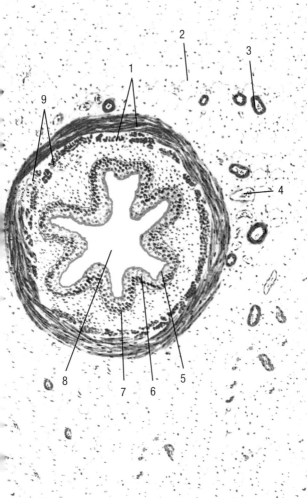

The Brain

Microscopic view

Inferior view - looking up onto the undersurface of the brain

Lateral view - looking at the side of the brain

Posterior view - looking at the back of the brain

Lateral view - showing the hidden GM

The brain consists of the CEREBRUM, CEREBELLUM, MIDBRAIN, and HIND BRAIN which leads to the SC.

The CEREBRUM overlies most of the brain and consists of 5 lobes named according to the bones which they underly, the hidden GM - the INSULA is buried under the overgrowth of the other cerebral lobes.

The outer GM is arranged as a series of folds to maximize the surface area: the gyri are the convex folds and the sulci, the fissures or grooves b/n them. They are named according to their anatomical position.

1   Frontal lobes - mainly for thinking & planning
2   Longitudinal fissure - Separates the 2 CHs
3   Parietal lobe - mainly for integration of sensory input
4   Parietal sulcus = Occipital fissure
5   Occipital lobe - for vision
6   Cerebellum
7   SC coming from the brainstem (Hindbrain)
8   Temporal lobe - mainly for language, memory & emotion
9   Lateral fissure = Sylvian fissure
10 Central sulcus = Central fissure
11 CH
12 Cerebellar hemisphere
13 Posterior lobe of the cerebellum
14 Vermis = (worm)
15 Folia - small gyri and sulci of the cerebellum
16 Pons = (bridge)
17 Infundibulum = (funnel) of the pituitary (removed)
18 Cranial Ns
19 Operculum - GM over the Insula
20 Insula = GM hidden under Cerebrum overgrowth

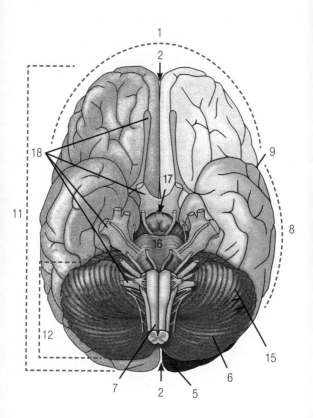

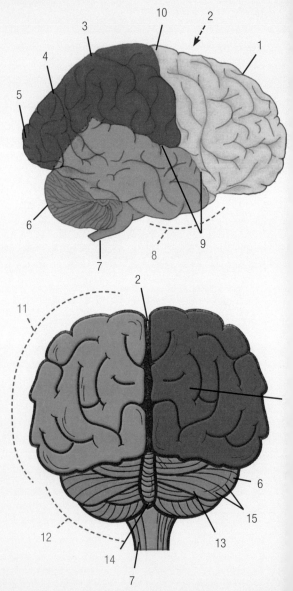

© A. L. Neill

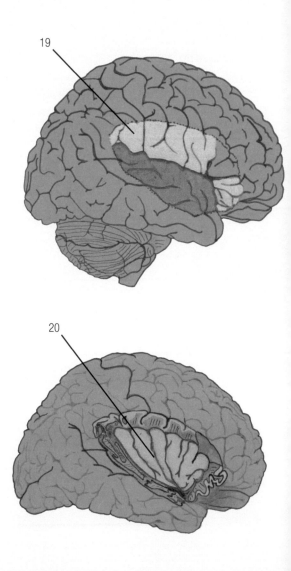

19

20

The Brain

Microscopic view
Median - midsagittal plane

1. Gyrus rectus – straight gyrus
2. Optic structures = CN II
3. Pituitary gland
4. IVth ventricle
5. Frontal lobe
6. Mammillary body
7. Pons
8. Olive
9. Hindbrain
10. SC + spinal canal
11. Temporal lobe
12. Cerebellum
13. Pineal body (= gland)
14. Lingual gyrus
15. Calcarine sulcus
16. Cuneus
17. Parieto-occipital sulcus
18. Precuneus
19. Post-central gyrus
20. Central sulcus
21. Paracentral gyrus = Precentral gyrus
22. Medical frontal = marginal gyrus
23. Thalamus + intermediate body
24. Fornix + Septum pellucidum
25. Minor gyri and sulci
26. Cingulum
27. Corpus callosum

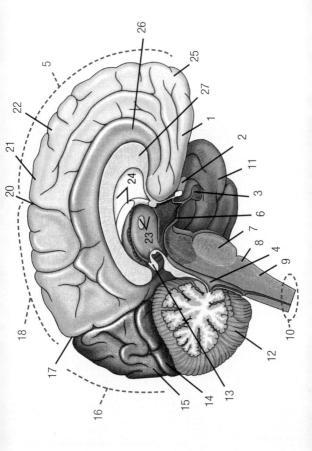

© A. L. Neill

The Brain

Macroscopic view

Superior - looking down on the brain from above

The Cerebrum is covered in GM with 4 major lobes and a covered area of GM - the Insula or 5th lobe.

1 FRONTAL LOBE
2 **OCCIPITAL LOBE**
3 **PARIETAL LOBE**
4 TEMPORAL LOBE
5 **INSULA**

Because of the overgrowth of the GM the brain creates additional area by forming large folds - GYRI (g) separated by fissures - SULCI (s)

A central sulcus = Rolandic fissure b/n the frontal and parietal lobes

B parieto-occipital sulcus

C preoccipital notch

D lateral sulcus = Sylvian fissure b/n the temporal and the frontal + parietal lobes

E stem of the lateral sulcus

L longitudinal suclus = longitudinal fissure b/n the R and L CH

further subdivided w/n the lobes by minor sulci

j lunate sulcus

h transverse occipital sulcus

i inferior temporal sulcus

l intra parietal sulcus

k associated rami of the lateral sulcus

1Ag pre-central gyrus MOTOR

2Ag post central gyrus SENSORY

2Ig inferior parietal gyrus (lobule)

2Sg superior parietal gyrus (lobule)

1Sg superior frontal gyrus

1Fg mid frontal gyrus

1Ig inferior frontal gyrus

4Dg superior temporal gyrus

4Ig inferior temporal gyrus

4Mg mid temporal gyrus

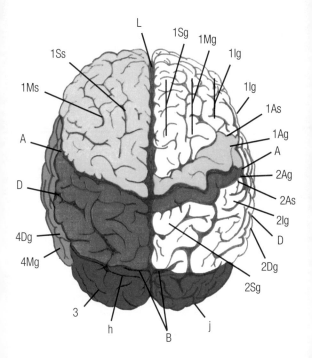

L

1Ss

1Ms

1Sg

1Mg

1Ig

1Ig

1As

A

1Ag

A

D

2Ag

2As

4Dg

2Ig

4Mg

D

3

2Dg

h

2Sg

B

j

Brain
Glia & BBB

Schema
LP of overall glia in the GM
HP of the BBB

The brain is a very protected organ forming its own environment via a special BBB and special supportive cells called glial cells. These cells interact with the meninges, neurons, BVs and influence their environment - helping with the neuron's health, nourishment, repair and ability to send and receive electrical signals.

1   BM of the endothelium - of the cerebral BV
2   foot process of the astrocyte
3   BM
4   glial limitans - formed from the subpial foot processes of the astrocytes - sealing the GM from the CSF surrounding the brain
5   astrocytes
6   digodendrocytes = Schwann cells in the CNS
7   neuron
8   microglia = fibroblast in the CNS
9   ependyma
10 ventricle
11 BV - note the BM is thickened and covered internally and externally
12 pericyte
13 sulcus
14 gyrus
15 pia mater
16 endothelium of the cerebral capillaries showing Tj

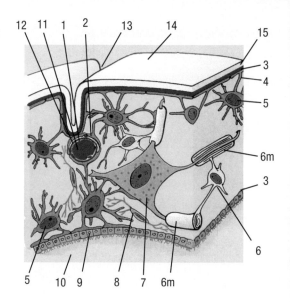

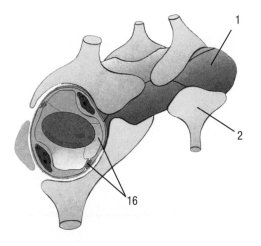

Brain
Neurons Cerebrum & Cerebellum

Schema

LP of overall neuronal arrangement of the cerebrum

LP of the overall neuronal arrangement of the cerebellum

HP of neuron types

The brain's major functioning cell is the neuron. There are a number of forms for these cells - some confined to the CNS which are often more branched and complex and some only found outside it, in the PNS. These neurons are arranged in layers in the GM of the cerebrum and although these layers vary in depth and content regionally, their basic form is maintained. The cerebellar layers are more rigidly maintained.

I	molecular layer
II	external granular layer
III	external pyramidal layer
IV	internal granular layer
V	internal pyramidal layer = ganglionic layer
VI	multiform cell layer = polymorphic layer
A	molecular layer
B	Purkinje cell layer
C	granule cell layer
WM	White matter note the of N impulses are bidirectional

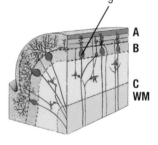

1	pyramidal cell	9	Purkinje cell
2	interneuron	10	bipolar neuron
3	axon	11	pseudobipolar cell
4	dendrite	12	motor neuron
5	cell bodies	13	autonomic neuron
6	Nissl bodies		p = pre-synaptic motor
7	smooth m		neuron
8	striated m generally skeletal m		q = post-synaptic motor neuron

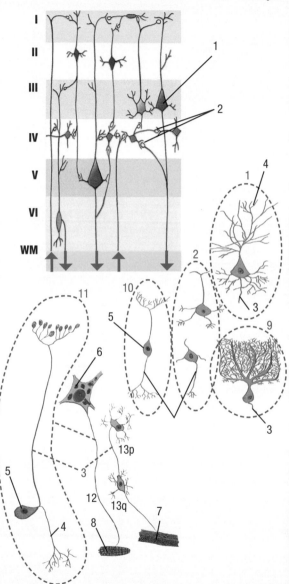

Colon = Large intestine (LI)

Macroscopic view

The colon or LI has 5 main parts if the caecum is included. It is part of the DT & 1.5m long. Its main function is to transport and prepare the remaining chyme for defecation. Bile salts are reabsorbed along with vitamin B_{12} which with water are the only materials resorbed in this area. It rings the abdominal cavity being fixed retroperitoneally along the sides. The transverse colon and sigmoid colon have their own mesenteries.

1. ileum
2. ileocaecal valve – site of vitamin B_{12} & bile resorption
3. vermiform appendix = appendix
4. caecum (5-7cm)
5. GALT
6. ascending colon = R sided colon (12cm) fixed to the post abdominal wall – no mesentery
7. hepatic flexure = R colic flexure
8. transverse Colon = horizontal colon (45cm) has a mesentery which allows movement
9. splenic flexure = L colic flexure – higher than the R - inf. to the spleen
10. appendices epiploicae – small fat filled tags - ↑ in size with ↑fat storage
11. taeniae coli – one of 3 discontinuous layers of longitudinal muscle in the LI
12. sigmoid colon = S – shaped colon (20-30cm) has a separate mesentery may store up to 2 kg of matter
13. rectum – fixed
14. anorectal junction
15. levator ani m
16. anus
17. internal semi-lunar valves
18. inner circular layer of the LI – continuous
19. mucosal surface

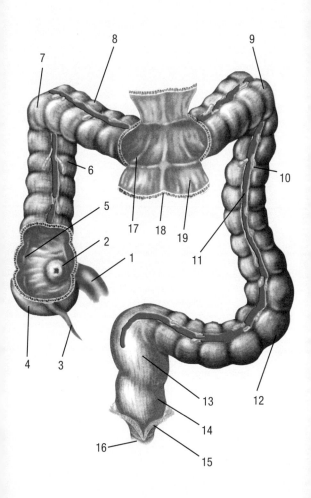

Digestive tract = DT

Schema

Macroscopic view - overview of the entire tract

The DT is the tract taken by food from the mouth to the anus. The main component is a long muscular tube which: transports, breaks up, digests & absorbs the food and liquids taken in from the mouth, before disposing of the remaining material and waste products of the body. The GIT describes the stomach to the colon inclusive. The GIT is 5m (20ft) long in life & may be stretched up to 9m (30ft) w/o muscle tone. Hs released from cells in the GIT to regulate the digestion process include: gastrin, secretin, cholecystokinin, and grehlin. They are mediated through either intracrine or autocrine mechanisms, located mainly in the epithelial lining of the DT.

1. oesophagus (10-14cm) a straight transport tube from mouth → stomach
2. changes from transport to digestion - gastro-oesophageal junction
3. stomach (volume up to 2 litres) acidic environment (ph1-4) digests food & kills bacteria, the mucosal lining needs to be protected from the acid with a thick mucus covering
4. pyloric sphincter divides the stomach & the duodenum regulating food entrance into the SI
5. duodenum 1st part of the SI = a 4 part tube – 25cm long, alkaline environment & site of entrance of bile and pancreatic enzymes
6. jejunum 2/5 of the total length of the SI & the main site of absorption - so large surface area of the mucosa for absorption
7. ileum 3/5 of the SI
   6 + 7 = SI
8. ileocaecal junction separates the SI & the LI via the ileocaecal valve, site of B_{12} and bile absorption
9. vermiform appendix – function? (AKA appendix)
10. caecum – storage sac of the LI
11. LI - main site of transport, water resorption & faecal concentration, minimal absorption
    H = haustrations = outpouchings in the wall where the longitudinal muscle is discontinuous - this allows for slower transit time and water retention
    T = taeniae coli, the discontinuous outer smooth muscle layer of the LI – storage site – minimal digestion, site of storage and faecal concentration

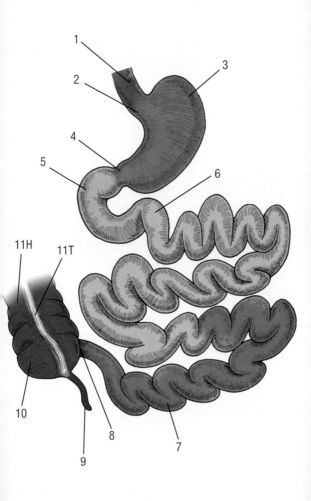

Digestive tract = DT

Schema

Comparison of layers on each segment

The DT tract shows regional variations which reflect the function of each segment, but the basic structure and layers are constant throughout.

A oesophagus

B stomach

C SI

D LI

   1 epithelial lining

   2 LP & a muscular layer muscularis mucosa

       1 + 2 = mucosa

   3 submucosa

   4 muscularis externa - with internal NS stimulated by ParaNS inner circular / outer longitudinal

   5 serosa ± mesentery

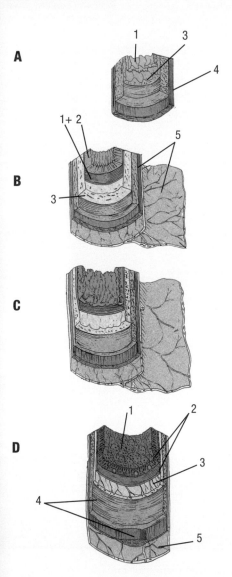

Digestive tract = DT

Schema
Comparison of segments

The DT tract shows regional variations particularly in the mucosal glands, lining epithelial layers and GALT (gut associated lymphoid tissue).

	REGION & FUNCTION	MUCOSA	SUBMUCOSA
A	**oesophagus** transport pH neutral	stratified squamous epi (i) glds+	glds ++ GALT +
B	**stomach** acidification digestion / liquification acid pH	epi - mucosal cells to coat and protect from acid - like goblet cells (ii), parietal cells = acid producing cells (iii), chief cells = pepsinogen enzyme producing cells (iv), endocrine cells (v) glds ++++ 3 regions cardiac, fundus, pyloris	GALT +
C	**SI** neutralization absorption alkaline pH	absorptive epi (vi) > goblet cells (vii) 3 regions duodenum jejunum, ileum, glds +++ villi ++++	glds ++ only in duodenum external glandular input from the pancreas & GB GALT +++++
D	**LI** water retrieval faecal formation pH varies	absorptive epi (vi) < goblet cells (vii) 5 parts caecum, ascending, transverse, descending, sigmoid	GALT +++

The appendix lies in the junction b/n SI & LI.

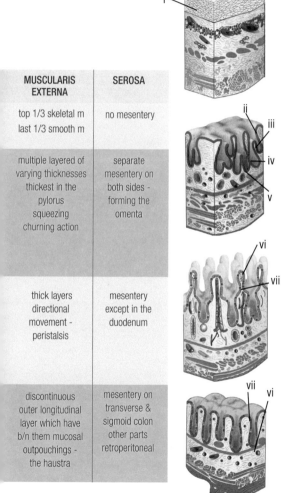

MUSCULARIS EXTERNA	SEROSA
top 1/3 skeletal m last 1/3 smooth m	no mesentery
multiple layered of varying thicknesses thickest in the pylorus squeezing churning action	separate mesentery on both sides - forming the omenta
thick layers directional movement - peristalsis	mesentery except in the duodenum
discontinuous outer longitudinal layer which have b/n them mucosal outpouchings - the haustra	mesentery on transverse & sigmoid colon other parts retroperitoneal

Digestive tract = DT

Histology
Junctional changes
LP H&E overview
oesophagus / stomach junction

The DT changes as it passes through its different regions with their specialized functions.

Between the oesophagus and the stomach the function changes from transport to digestion, hence the lining epithelium changes from stratified to simple columnar.

1   oesophagus
2   stomach
3   stratified squamous epithelium
4   LP
5   oesophageal mucosal glands
6   exocrine ducts
7   muscularis mucosa
8   submucosal glands
9   submucosa - also LP
10 muscularis externa
11 gastric pits - with mucosal glands in the cardiac area of the stomach
12 gastric glands deeper and with specialized cells in the fundus area
13 parietal cells - acid producing cells
14 chief cells = peptic cells = zymogen cells - produce pepsinogen enzyme precursor for digestion
15 mucous cells to protect it from acid auto digestion coating the stomach surface

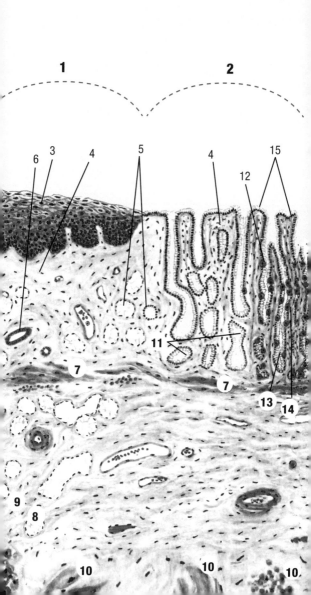

Digestive tract = DT

Histology
Junctional changes
LP H&E overview
pylorus / duodenum junction

The DT changes as it passes through its different regions with their specialized functions.

Between the pyloris of the stomach and the duodenum the function changes from gross material digestion in an acid environment which has liquefied the material (chyme) to further digestion & absorption in an alkaline environment.

1 pyloris (stomach)
2 duodenum (SI)
3 gastric mucosal epithelium
4 LP
5 mucosal ridges - rugae (in the stomach)
6 gastric mucosal glands - these are commoner at the cardiac and pyloric ends of the stomach
7 muscularis mucosa - moves up into the villi in the duodenum
8 submucosa - also LP
9 muscularis externa - multiple layers of smooth m in the stomach but only 2 in the duodenum
10 serosa
11 duodenal glands (Brünner's glands)
12 lymphoid follicle of GALT
13 intestinal gland
14 villi - structured folds in the SI - these are low & numerous in the duodenum, highest in the jejunum and lower and less numerous in the ileum
15 goblet cell
16 intestinal absorptive cells

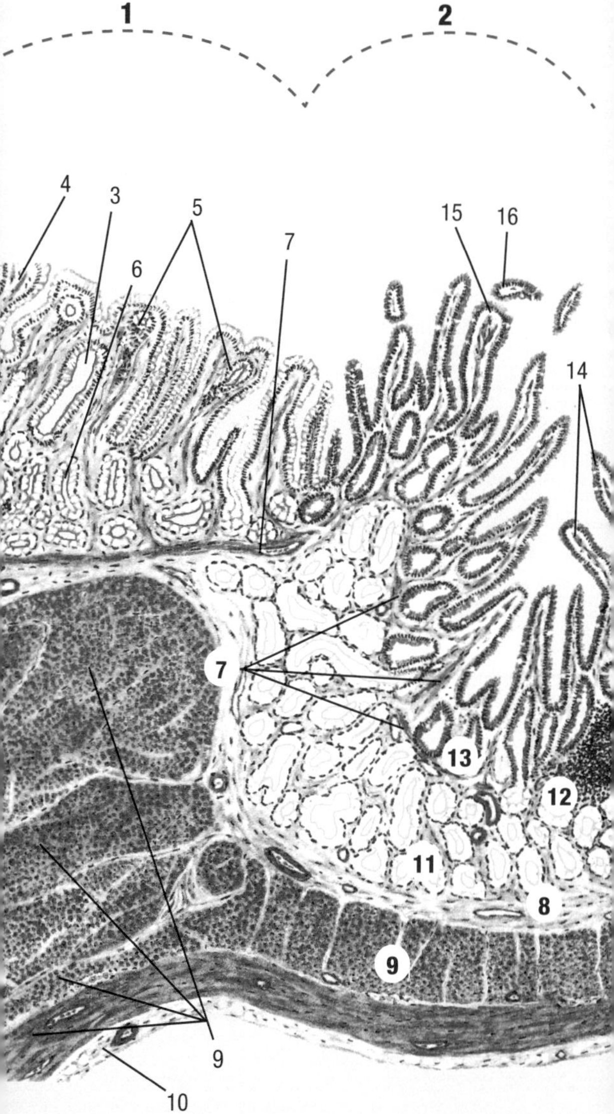
1
2
4
3
5
6
7
15
16
14
7
13
12
11
8
9
9
10

Digestive tract = DT

Histology
Junctional changes
LP H&E overview
anorectal junction

The DT changes as it passes through its different regions with their specialized functions.

Between the anus - the lower end of the LI and the rectum the function changes from transport, water resorption and involuntary peristalsis to extrusion. The mucus covered stool has been moulded and stored in the LI to take on a suitable shape and consistency for defecation. As with the oesopho-gastric junction the BS also changes from the portal LP system to the HP systemic BF and build up here will result in engorgement of the BVs which may then protrude as haemorrhoids. The movement of the mass also changes so that the muscle is replaced with skeletal muscle to allow it to be under voluntary control.

1 anus
2 rectum
3 stratified squamous epithelium
4 LP
5 internal haemorrhoidal plexus of BVs
6 lymphoid nodules of GALT
7 EAS - skeletal m
8 levator ani - skeletal mu
9 IAS - skeletal m
10 submucosa - also LP
11 muscularis mucosa
12 intestinal mucoid glands
13 mucosa LP
14 columnar epithelium with many goblet cells

　　　　　　　　　　　　　　© A. L. Neill

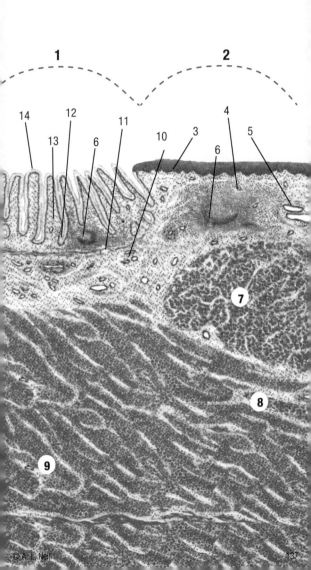

© A. L. Neill

Ear

Macroscopic view
Coronal plane

The ear has 3 main components - the outer ear - which is the external part of the organ; the middle ear and the inner ear concerned with balance and sense of position, as well as hearing.

1   cochlea
2   eustachian tube = auditory tube
3   round window
4   stapes
5   incus
6   malleus
7   CN VII = Facial N
8c Cochlear N – part of CN VIII
8v Vestibular N part of CN VIII
9   Tympanic membrane
10 IAM
11 EAM
12 Pinna

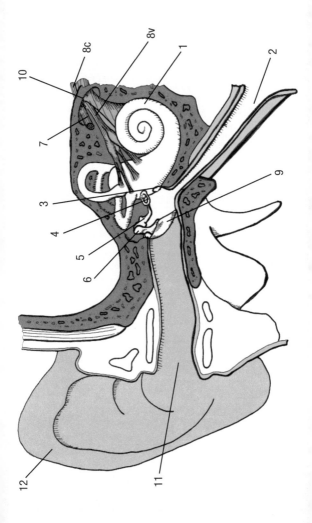

Ear
Middle & Inner ears

Macroscopic view

The "ear" has at least 2 functions. As well as hearing, the ear is also responsible for balance and body position. The external ear ends at the level of the tympanic membrane (2) and the inner ear begins beyond the ear's tympanic cavity with the middle ear in b/n. The function of hearing and balance are intimately related and share a common CN which has 2 parts. The cochlea is a fluid filled tube which decreases in volume along its length, which is coiled and has membrane windows at either end for the transmission of sound vibrations. Hair cells detect these along the cochlea length and their responses are conveyed to the dendrites of the cochlear N (part of the CN VIII).

1 EAM - leading in from the auricle & ending at the...

2 tympanic membrane

3 auditory ossicles
   i malleus
   ii incus
   iii stapes

4 semicircular canal in the bony duct which lies in the...

5 Temporal bone

6 crista ampullaris

7 facial N = CN VII

8 vestibular N = part of CN VIII

9 CN VIII = vestibulocochlear N

10 IAM

11 cochlea

12 part of the bony labyrinth

13 auditory tube AKA Eustachian tube AKA pharyngotympanic tube – (35mm long) note the wall changing from bone 1/3 to cartilage – empties into the inf. nasal concha & regularises P in the inner & middle ears

14 cochlear duct

15 saccule

16 internal jugular v

17 tympanic cavity

18 oval window

19 round window

20 utricle

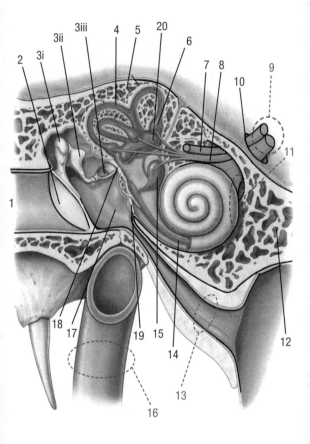

Ear
Cochlea

Schema
cochlea cross-section LP
cochlea - individual section MP
cochlea - organ of Corti HP

The cochlea is the organ of hearing and lies in the inner ear. It relies upon the movement of lymph through the fluid filled cochlear canal.

A Scala Vestibuli

B Scala Media

C Scala Tympani

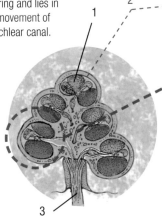

1   helicotrema
2   cochlear duct
3   CN VIII = vestibulocochlear N
4   vestibular membrane = Reissner's membrane
5   spiral limbus on the osseous spiral lamina
6   dendrite of the cochlear N (part of CN VIII)
7   basilar membrane
8   spiral organ of Corti
9   spiral prominence
10 stria vascularis
11 spiral lig
12 tectorial membrane
13 hair cells
14 border cell
15 phalangeal cell
16 pillar cells
17 Bottcher's cells
18 Claudius cells
i = inner   o = outer

© A. L. Neill

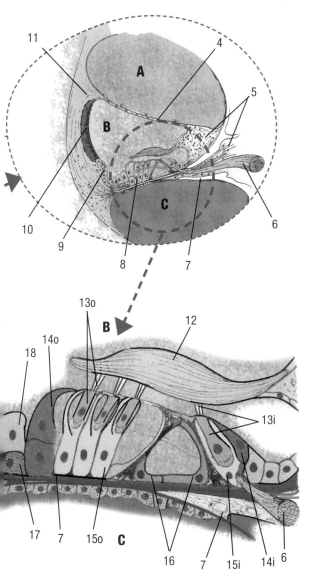

Ear - cochlea

Histology
LP H&E overview of the components

The cochlea is the organ of hearing of the inner ear. It is a spiraled hollow conical chambre of bone (A) with a central modiolus (B) for signal transmission via the N. Vibrations from the middle ear windows are transmitted along the cochlea hollow and through its 3 scalae - or divisions of the hollow chambre, which becomes confluent in the helicotrema.

These 3 sections are filled with fluids and separated by membranes upon which lie specialized hair cells - forming the organ of Corti. It is this organ that interprets the vibrations into elecrtical impulses - later "heard" as sounds in the brain.

1 helicotrema
2 scala vestibuli = vestibular duct
3 scala media = cochlear duct
4 scala tympani = tympanic duct
5 outer bony wall of the cochlea
6 spiral lig
7 spiral ganglion
8 cochlear N (part of CN VIII)
9 basilar membrane
10 tectorial membrane
11 organ of Corti
12 vestibular membrane (Reissner's membrane)
13 osseous spiral lamina

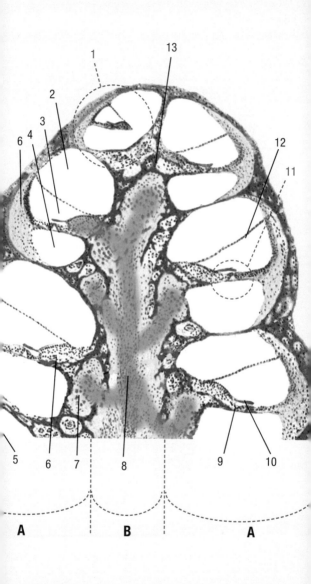

Ear
Cochlear & Vestibular canals

Schema
Overview of the bony (A) & membranous (B) labyrinths and cochlear (Cc) & vestibular canals (Cv)
Schema of the hair cells

Balance, body position and hearing are determined by the movement of the sensory hair cells of the semicircular canals of the inner ear. The canals are placed at R angles to each other, so movement in any direction moves the hair cells, which generates electrical E and sensory input.

1 semi-circular canals-- anterior, posterior & lateral...

2 membrane windows r = round / o = oval

3 saccule - r = recess for this structure / m = macula of

4 utricle - r = recess for this swelling / m = macula of

5 cochlea d = duct

6 endolymph endolymphatic
d = duct
s = sac

7 space around the canals in the bony labyrinth

8 crista ampullaris

9 organ of Corti

10 otoliths

11 cupola

12 dendrites of the vestibular N

13 hair cells
i = type 1 - pyriform & totally enclosed in 1 main dendrite
ii = type 2 - cylindrical with several N ending attachments

14 supportive cells

15 kinocilia - extremely long stiff cytoplasmic extension longer than...

16 stereocilia

17 BM

18 dendrites

19 efferent Ns

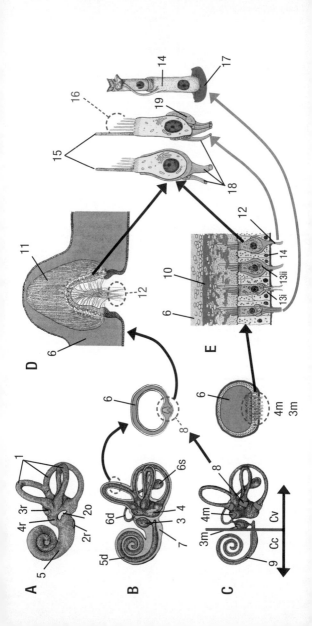

Eye

Macroscopic view
surface anatomy & features
Anterior - face on

1   eyebrow
2   upper eyelid orbital part
3   palpebral sulcus i = inferior, s = superior
4   upper eyelid tarsal part
5   angle of the eye L = lateral, m = medial
    in b/n the palpebral fissure 5f (where the upper & lower lids meet)
6   nasal jugal sulcus
7   eyelashes
8   malar sulcus = lateral sulcus
9   iris
10 pupil

11 sclera = bulbar conjunctiva
12 papilla lacrimalis (raised surface)
13 punctum lacrimale (opening for tear duct)
14 caruncula lacrimalis = lacrimal caruncle – (tear duct)
15 lacus lacrimalis
16 plica semilunaris
17 palpebral conjunctiva
18 lower lid margins (ant & post)
19 tarsal glands and openings
20 inf fornix of the conjunctiva

21 branches of posterior conjunctival arteries
22 tarsal plate (lower is much thinner 22L)
23 upper lid margins (ant & post)

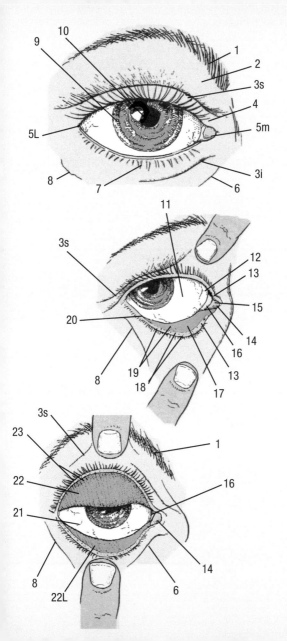

Eye
Lacrimal apparatus

Macroscopic view

The lacrimal apparatus consists of the lacrimal glands - small almond shaped glands mainly found in the upper outer corner of each eye socket - the lacrimal fossa, with smaller palpebral parts found along the inside of the eyelid; and the ducts to drain their secretions. The glands form tears which may be stimulated by physical or emotional factors; neural input is via the ANS. They also lubricate the eye in association with the tarsal glds.

1   lacrimal gld (main orbital part)
2   secretory ducts
3   superior & inferior canaliculi
4   common canaliculus
5   lacrimal sac
6   naso-lacrimal duct cell membrane = CM
7   inf. nasal concha
8   inf. nasal meatus
9   nasal cavity
10 superior & inferior lacrimal puncta

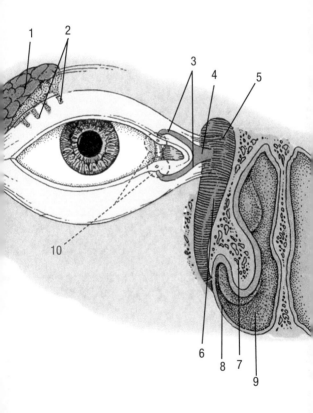

Eye
Eyelid - relationship with eyeball

Macroscopic view
Parasagittal

The eyelid passes across the eyeball cleaning and lubricating it with each blink, which occurs on average 4 - 6X/min - slower in infants and faster in adolescents. The lacrimal & tarsal glds combine to form the lubrication & prevent evaporation from the corneal surface, which is a dry T internally and so needs to be lubricated via its surface. The amount of secretion ↓ with age.

1. lacrimal gld
   a = accessory glds - may be found along the eyelid
2. superior tarsal m = muscle of Müller
3. subcut fat - varies with ethnicity
4. CT fibres
5. orbicularis oculi m
6. skin of the eyelid
7. tarsal ligs
8. tarsal plate
9. tarsal gld AKA meibomian gld AKA sebaceous gld (of the eye)
10. eyelash
11. sebaceous gld (of Moll)
12. conjunctiva - palpabral and bulbar
13. cornea
14. anterior chambre
15. iris
16. lens
17. zonula fibres - suspend the lens
18. ciliary body - produces fluid for the anterior chambre
19. vitreous chambre
20. sclera
21. conjunctival fornix

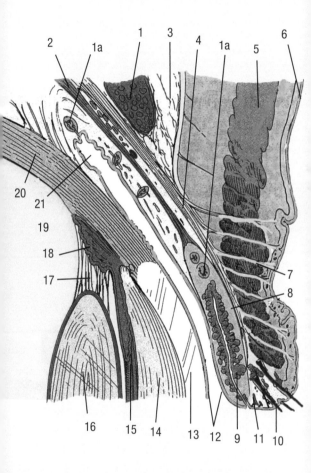

Eyelid

Histology
LP H&E overview showing most structures

The eyelid protects and facilitates lubrication of the eye. The lamina propria of the subcut. T has a specialist CT dense structure, the tarsus which maintain a stiff convex curve as the eyelid moves over the eyeball surface with blinking.

1 hair follicle
2 adipose cells
3 sebaceous gld of the follicle
4 epidermis
5 sweat glds
6 dermis = CT
7 orbicularis oculi m
8 eyelash hair follicles
9 ciliary m = muscle of Rollen
10 tarsal
    d = duct
    g = gland
11 sweat glds - near eyelashes = glds of Moll
12 tarsus = tarsal plate
13 palpebral conjunctiva
14 BVs
15 lymphatic tissue
16 superior tarsal muscle = muscle of Müller

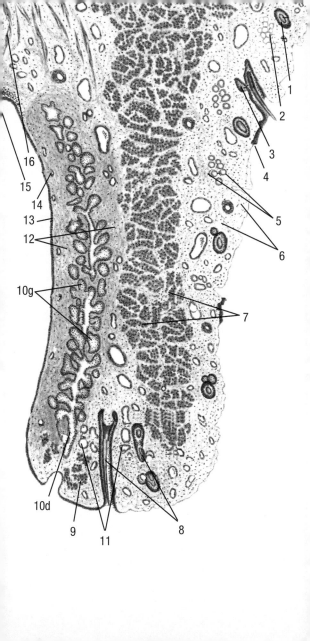

Eye
Lacrimal gland

Histology
MP H&E

This gland lubricates the cornea of the eye, hence the glands present are seromucoid and secrete along the ducts as well as in the acini. It protects the eye from both dryness & infection.

1. myoepithelial cells surrounding the glands
2. adipose cells
3. interlobular excretory duct
4. acini
5. a & v
6. CT septa
7. N

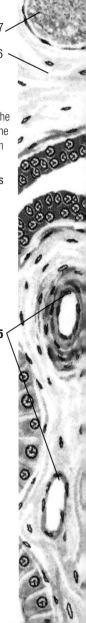

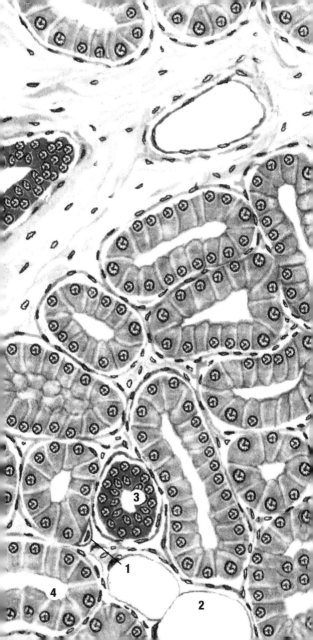

Eyeball

Macroscopic view

superior view skull and brain removed

deep and superficial dissections noting detailed musculature and NS

The eye is a complex organ - it sits in its bony socket with numerous CNs supplying its surrounding muscles and the retina - for sight.

1 rectus m
2 Optic N - CN II & chiasma
3 Oculomotor N - CN III
4 Trochlear N - CN IV
5 Trigeminal N - CN V
6 Abducent N - CN VI
7 lacrimal gland
8 oblique m
9 eyeball - globe

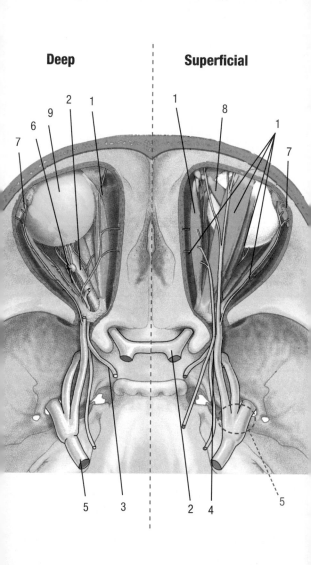

Deep

Superficial

Eyeball

Histology
LP H&E overview showing most structures

The eyeball is the organ of vision. It sits snugly in the eye socket surrounded by loose areolar T to allow for free movement and has a posterior opening to allow for the passage of BVs and the optic N (CN II).

1. cornea
2. pupil
3. anterior (aqueous humour) and posterior chambers of the eye
4. iris
5. ciliary processes from the cilary m
6. suspensory lig = zonular fibres
7. choroid
8. retina
9. optic papilla – blind spot
10. optic N (CN II)
11. macula fovea – focus site
12. vitreous humour – gel like material in the eye should be adherent only at the macula, optic N & ora serrata
13. sclera – white of the eye made of dense CT
14. ora serrata – small section (8mm) of the epithelium b/n the ciliary body and the retina which secretes nutrients into the humours of the eye to supply the internal structures
15. limbus
16. lens

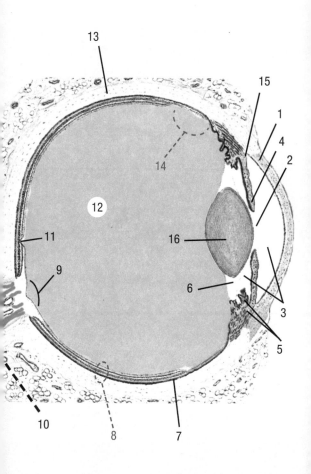

Eyeball – components
Cornea & Retina

Histology

LP corneal layers & retinal layers overview

The eyeball is a highly stratified organ - the structured layers facilitate the passage and focus of incident light in its anterior region via the cornea & lens and interpret the image via photosensitive T on its back surface - the retina.

A anterior limiting membrane = Bowman's membrane

B corneal stroma – substantia propria = densely packed lattice CT

C posterior limiting membrane = Descemet's membrane

D eyeball contents including lens & vitreous humour

E retina

F choroid

G sclera

L direction of incident light

1 stratified squamous corneal epithelium

2 BM

3 fibroblasts & fibrocytes

4 collagen fibres-type VIII

5 simple cuboidal epithelium - endothelium

6 inner limiting membrane

7 ganglion layer

8 inner & outer plexiform layers

9 inner & outer nuclear layers

10 rods & cones – cells of vision

11 pigmented epithelium

12 BVs

13 melanocytes

14 collagen fibres

© A. L. Neill

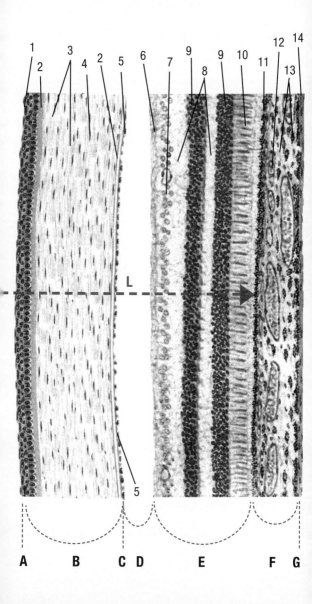

Eyeball - components
Retina

Micro Schema

The retina has 9 distinct layers, seen clearly in sections and they are due to the highly organized nature of this specialized structure.

These are in order from the retinal surface to the base:

ILM internal limiting membrane

NFL nuclear fibre layer

GCL ganglion cell layer

IPL inner plexiform layer

INL inner nuclear layer

OPL outer plexiform layer

ONL outer nuclear layer

ELM external limiting membrane

P photoreceptors + pigmented epithelium intimately connected

L direction of incident light

1. ganglion cell
2. amarcrin cell
3. bipolar cell
4. horizontal cell
5. photoreceptive cell
6. specialized endings
    - c = cones
    - r = rods
7. pigmented epithelial cells
8. Müller cells - supporting the specialist cells

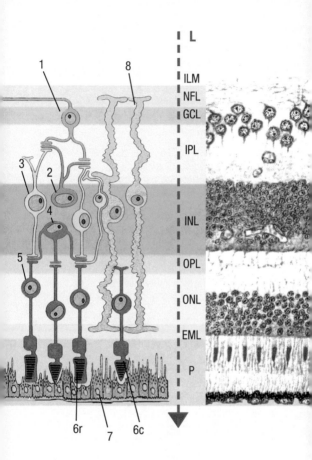

L

ILM
NFL
GCL

IPL

INL

OPL

ONL

EML

P

Eyeball - components
Iris & Lens

Schema

The amount of light entering the eye is controlled by a circular muscle, the iris which determines the size of the pupil. It is then focused on the back of the eye by the lens. Depending upon the distance of the object from the eye, the lens will become more or less convex, determined by the ciliary m so that it is focused on the back of the eye. Like all things in the eye these actions are highly coordinated. The cells of the lens grow from the equator down the anterior surface of the lens and produce a lengthening fibre as they progress.

1　germinal zone - on the lens equator
2　lens capsule - made of the BM - fibrous sac
3　lens fibre
4　germinal epithelium - generates the lens fibre and moves down the ant surface of the lens
5　pupillary margin
6　melanocyte
7　ridges and grooves in the iris b/n cells
8　fibroblast
9　macrophage
10　muscles of the iris
　　　d = dilator pupillae
　　　s = sphincter pupillae
11　myoepithelial cells - in contact with the mu
12　pigmented epithelial cells - sitting on the BM and growing downwards
13　BM - of the iris

L = direction of incident light

© A. L. Neill

Gall Bladder (GB)

Macroscopic view

The GB holds the excess bile produced by the liver. It releases this into the duodenum when stimulated. Bile from the liver moves down the hepatic ducts until stopped at the duodenal papilla, where by retrograde flow, it fills the fundus of the GB. The bile is released along with the pancreatic secretions to aid digestion, fat emulsion and absorption.

1   hepatic ducts L = left / R = right
2   common hepatic duct
3   Heister's valve
4   GB duct
5   common bile duct
6   pancreatic duct
7   opening of the pancreatic duct (into the common bile duct)
8   major duodenal papilla = Papilla of Vater (in the descending duodenum)
9   LN in the duodenum
10 plicae circulares of the Duodenum
11 serosa – capsule of the GB
12 fundus of the GB
13 mucosa
14 folds in the GB
15 body of the GB
16 neck of the GB

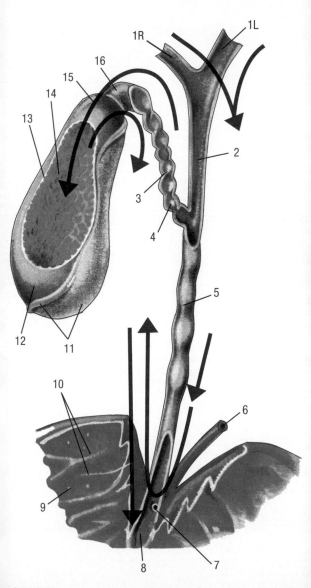

Gall Bladder

Histology

LP H&E overview

The gall bladder stores and concentrates the bile produced by the liver. It releases this into the DT for fat digestion when stimulated.

1 large mucosal folds
2 arteriole & venule in mucosa
3 smooth m layers spiral orientation (much as in the urinary bladder)
4 a & v of the capsule
5 mesothelium of the serosa
6 Ns
7 CT of the capsule
8 elastic fibres
9 crypts - diverticulae of the mucosa
10 BM
11 mucosal folds
12 polysaccharide coating on the lining columnar epithelium

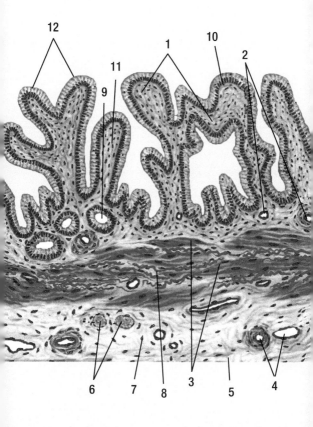

Heart

Macroscopic view

Pericardial sinuses - showing vessels entering - heart removed

Anterior - external surfaces

Posterior (diaphragmatic surface)

The heart pumps the blood around the body in 2 separate circulations - one at a LP through the lungs - the pulmonary circulation - and the other at HP around the body - the systemic circulation. It is a highly muscular organ and consists of 4 chambers. Blood is received from veins by the auricles - passes through the valves to the muscular ventricles, where it is pushed out via arteries.

1 L carotid artery
2 L subclavian artery
3 ligamentum arteriosum
4 L pulmonary artery L & R
5 pericardium
6 L auricle
7 L coronary artery
   a = ant. interventricular
   c = circumflex
   p = post. interventricular artery
8 great cardiac vein
9 LV
10 RV
11 IVC
12 small cardiac vein
13 RA
14 R coronary artery
   m = middle cardiac vein
15 R auricle
16 SVC
17 R brachiocephalic trunk
18 pulmonary veins L & R
19 coronary sinus
20 middle cardiac vein
21 apex of the heart
22 aorta
   a = ascending /
   r = arch / t = thoracic
23 pulmonary trunk
24 sinuses
   o = oblique
   t = transverse

© A. L. Neill

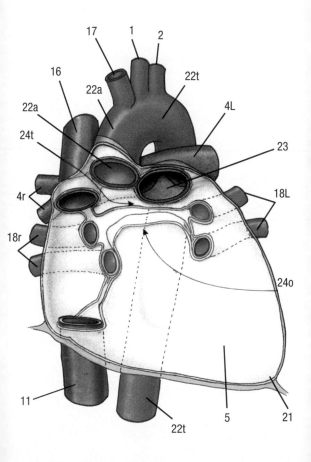

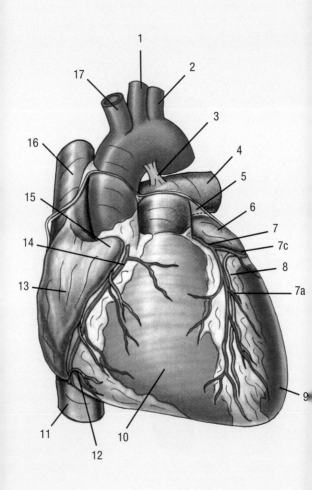

© A. L. Neill

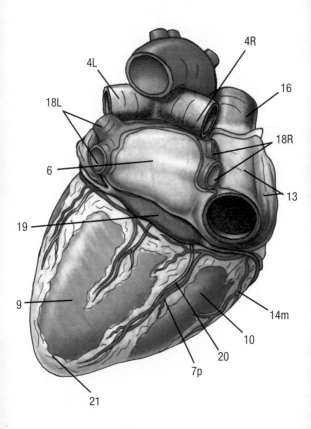

4R

4L

18L

16

6

18R

13

19

9

14m

10

20

7p

21

Heart

Macroscopic view
Anterior surface cutaway to see the 4 internal chambres

1 aortic arch
2 L pulmonary arteries
3 L pulmonary veins
4 LA
5 mitral valve = bicuspid valve
6 aortic valve - semilunar cusps
7 papillary muscles
8 interventricular septum
9 RV wall
10 chordae tendineae (attached to 7)
11 tricupsid valve
12 IVC
13 RA
14 pulmonary valve
15 pulmonary trunk arterial
16 SVC
17 ligamentum arteriosum

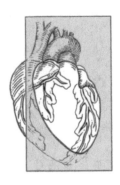

© A. L. Neill

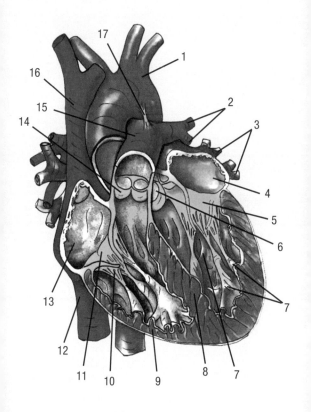

Kidneys

Macroscopic view

R kidney - sectioned in planes to show internal structures - capsule removed.

Paired kidneys in the abdomen ant. & post. view - note the capsule has been completely removed from the R kidney & partially removed from the L.

Due to the liver the R kidney sits lower than the L.

The kidneys are small paired encapsulated organs which sit on the back wall of the abdomen. They produce urine from filtering the blood, taking 20% of the CO. They determine the BP and the body's hydration. They have a cortex, medulla and pelvis with the urine draining through to the ureter and down to the bladder. Blood vessels enter and leave via the hilum.

1 renal column
2 cortex
3 medulla - pyramid
4 arcuate a
5 radial a & v
6 calices
  a = major
  m = minor
  p = pelvis - coalescing of all the calices
7 ureter (& BVs)
8 pelvic fat
9 hilum
10 fibrous capsule
11 renal vessels
  a = artery
  ap = polar arteries - these are variations appearing in 1/3 of patients v = vein

12 renal poles
  i = inferior
  s = superior
13 renal margins
  L = lateral
  m = medial
14 aorta - abdominal
15 IVC
16 mesenteric vessels inf. & superior
17 intercostal a
18 adrenal a
19 perseverance of the foetal lobules of the kidney - these show variation

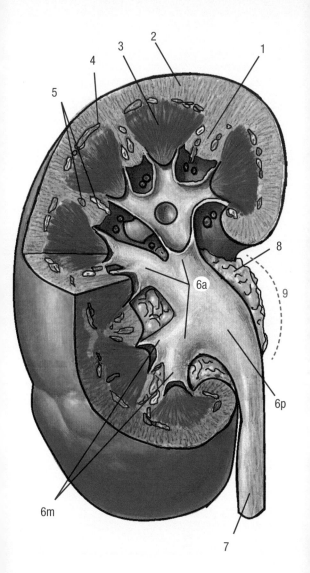

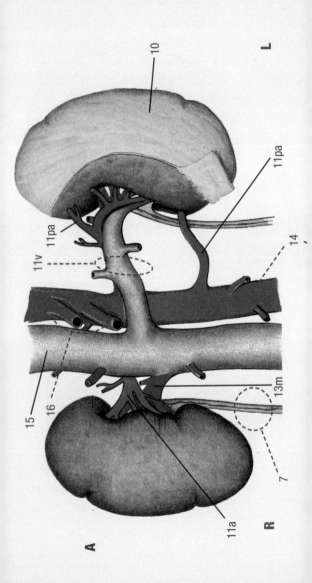

© A. L. Neill

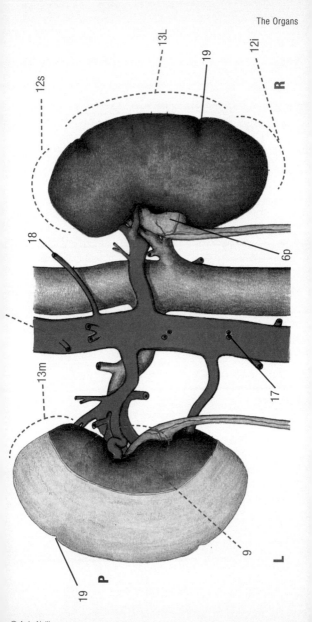

12s

13L

19

12i

R

18

6p

13m

17

9

P

19

L

© A. L. Neill

Kidney
Renal Corpuscle

Histology
HP H&E - showing most of the basic structures
HP Mallory's trichrome stain - to demonstrate reticular fibres & BM

The kidney functions to filter the B, eliminating wastes but conserving certain ions, proteins & water. The first step in this process is to push the fluid component through a knot of capillaries - the glomerulus - at ↑ P and capture it in a surrounding capsule. The whole structure is the renal corpuscle, the filtering unit of the nephron. There are approx. 1 million in each kidney, some located superficially in the cortex & others in the corticomedullary junction. The nephrons of these glomeruli determine the concentration of the urine with their long renal loops – (loops of Henle).

1 renal capsule (Bowman's capsule) outer (parietal) & inner (visceral) layers

    s = capsular space

2 PCT

3 glomerular capillaries

4 mesangial cells in the glomerulus

5 poles of the glomerulus

    u = urinary pole

    v = vascular pole

6 juxtaglomerular apparatus = macula densa (m) + juxtaglomerular cells (j)

7 BV - afferent & efferent arterioles

8 DCT

9 collecting duct

10 BM

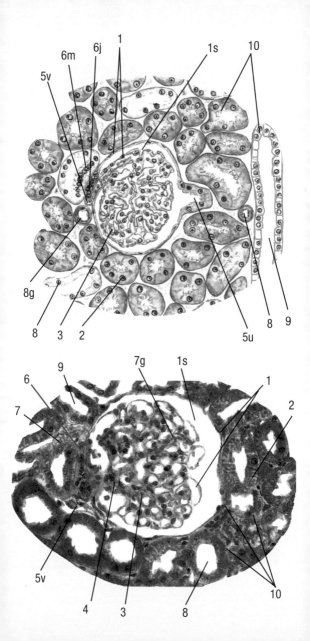

Kidney – functioning unit
Nephron

Schema

Order of tubules from the glomerulus

The kidney's primary function is the selected filtration of the blood fluid contents. The main functioning unit for this is the nephron. B is passed at a high pressure through a knot of capillaries (1) and the fluid collected in the surrounding capsule (2). After passing through a series of tubules (3) which alters its composition - it is collected (4) and forms the urine.

1   renal capillaries

   a - afferent - capillaries entering the glomerulus

   e - efferent - capillaries leaving the glomerulus

   g - glomerular capillaries - w/in the capsule

2   glomerular capsule = Bowman's capsule, fluid from the capillaries is collected here passing to the...

3   renal tubules

   d - DCT - closest to the collecting ducts -
   in the renal cortex

   L - loop tubules = Loop of Henle - thick and thin
   segments - thin as it descends into the renal pelvis
   - thickening as it joins the other tubular segments -
   in the renal medulla

   p - PCT - closest to the
   glomerulus - in the renal cortex

4   collecting ducts - feeding into the renal pelvis & ureter

5   renal venules

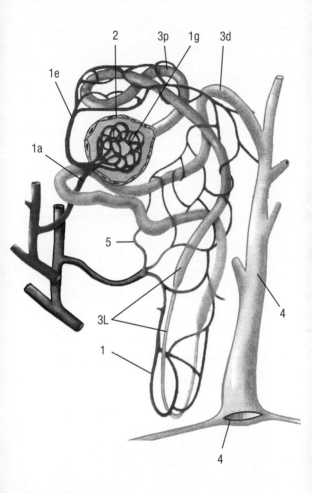

3p   3L   3d   1   4

Kidney

Nephron - components

Schema
Renal Corpuscle - Glomerulus + Capsule

A Mesangial cell & Capillaries

B PCT

The renal corpuscle is a HP vascular filter - arterioles enter the corpuscle to become glomerular capillaries. Their thicker walls are associated with muscle - like cells - the mesangial cells. The exiting BV is also an arteriole. The pressure of the afferent arteriole is highly regulated by the juxtaglomerular & macula densa cells, and this determines the amount and type of filtrate captured in the Bowman's capsule. The glomerular capillaries are fenestrated i.e. they have windows of CM only sections to allow for maximum fluid flow with minimum protein loss.

1 renal arterioles
   a - afferent - entering the glomerulus
   e - efferent - leaving the glomerulus
2 glomerular capsule = Bowman's capsule
   o = outer parietal layer - composed of flattened epithelial cells with Tj
   p = inner layer composed of podocytes - epithelial cells with modified foot processes (10)
3 DCT
   d = modified macula densa cells
4 glomerular capillaries
5 contractile cells
   s = smooth muscle cells of the arterioles
   m = mesangial cells of the glomerulus

6 BM - under every epithelial & endothelial layer
7 glomerular endothelial cells
   f = fenestrations
8 endothelial cells of the arterioles
9 juxtaglomerular cells
10 pedicles
11 matrix surrounding the mesangial cells
12 mv
13 cell borders / channels b/n cells - to allow facilitated passage of substances
14 basolateral channels creating elaborate canals b/n & w/n cells
15 mitochondria - lodged in and around these channels

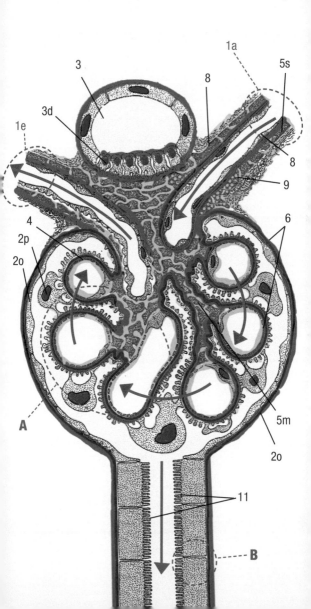

A

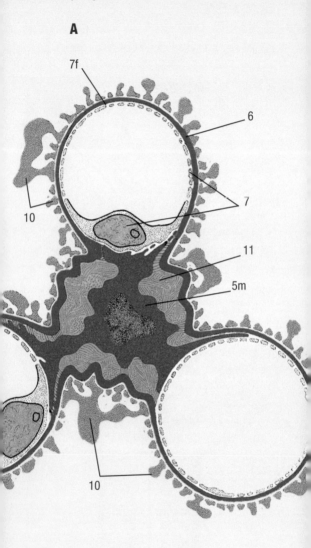

B

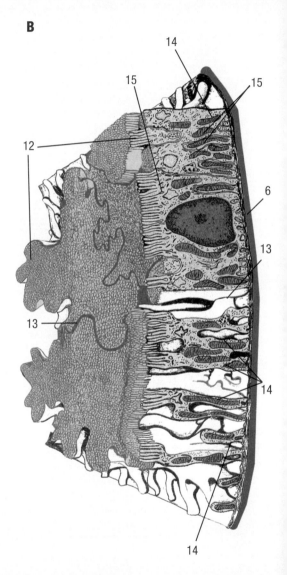

Liver

Macroscopic view

Anterior - in situ lying beneath the diaphragm
Inferior - reflected view i.e. liver lifted up in situ

The liver is an encapsulated organ and occupies most of the RUQ. It is the largest internal organ weighing up to 2kg and is suspended from the diaphragm by several ligaments. BVs from the GIT transport the highly nutrient-filled blood to this organ before going to the systemic BS. This portal BF is then combined with the hepatic BVs and empties into the IVC. Hence any toxins, medications or other substances are exposed to this filter and maybe altered deactivated or denatured before entering the systemic BS. The slow flow at low pressure of the B through the sinusoids allows for extensive exposure to the liver cells. There are 4 lobes anatomically but only 2 functionally, supplied by the R & L branches of the hepatic a.

1　main liver lobes L & R
2　diaphragm
3　falciform lig
4　ligamentum teres = round lig
5　gallbladder
6　quadrate lobe
7　porta hepatis
8　division b/n R & L lobes
9　caudate lobe
10　IVC
11　bare area on the superior liver surface
12　coronal lig

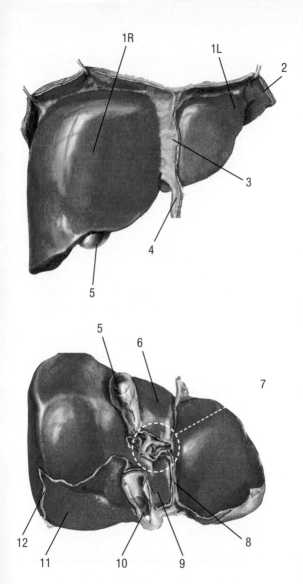

Liver

Histology

LP Mallory-Azan stain for CT - showing most of the basic structures

A = acinus - divided into 3 zones - zone 1 being the most oxygenated region, zone 3 being the least

L = lobule - hexagon ringed by CT septa

The liver is the biggest internal organ of the body with the structural unit of the Lobule and a functional unit of the Acinus. This is important in considering liver disease partic in CCF where the distance from oxygenated B becomes an important consideration, and determines the patterns of a developing cirrhosis.

1   central vein accepts the B from the portal triad (3)
2   walls of hepatocytes - liver parenchymal cells
3   portal triad containing...
4   hepatic arteriole - blood flows to the central vein
5   **bile ductule -** bile flows to the portal triad
6   **hepatic portal venule -** blood flows to the central vein
7   interlobular septum

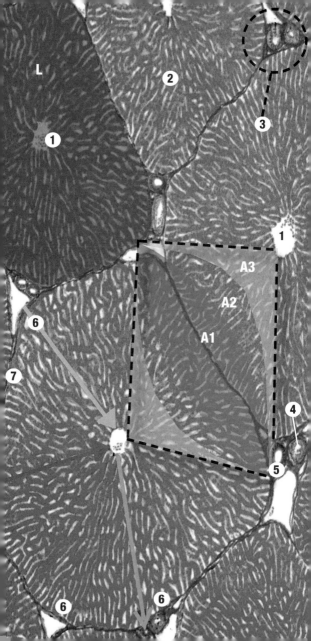

Liver

Histology
MP H&E to show basic cell types in the liver parenchyma
MP Reticular stain - to show fibrillar support in the liver
HP PAS stain to show glycogen storage in the hepatocytes
The liver has a number of functions and this is reflected in its many different cells. Ito cells: generating and supporting the reticular fibre structure; Kupffer cells phagocytose misshapen & old RBCs and bacteria; endothelial cells which line the sinusoids & hepatocytes which make up the bulk of the organ, which synthesize proteins, metabolise & detoxify substances.

1   portal vein
2   collagen fibres of the interlobular septum
3   sinusoid space
4   reticular fibes in sinusoids
5   hepatocyte walls of cells, some are binucleate & actively mitosing (others undergoing apoptysis)
6   collagen CT of the central vein
7   lumen of central vein
8   bile duct in portal triad
9   BM
10 endothelial cells of the sinusoids
11 Küpffer cells - the phagocytic cells of the liver
12 RBCs and PMNs in the sinusoids
13 glycogen stores in the hepatocytes
14 Ito cells - fibroblasts of the liver

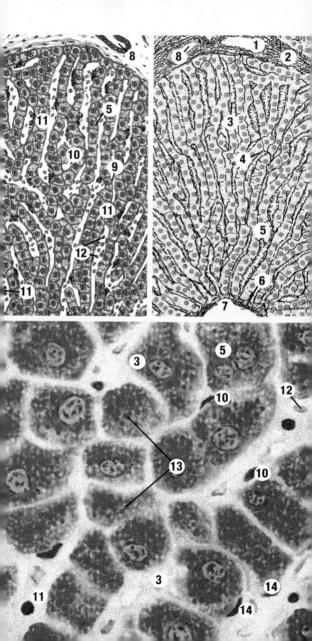

Liver

Schema
LP of liver lobule
HP of portal triad

The liver structurally is arranged in an hexagon formation of lobules, each with a central vein, and portal triads at the corners of the hexagon. The central veins and hence the lobules are connected by the sublobular intercalated veins which drain directly into the IVC.

1 portal triad
2 capillaries
3 terminal hepatic arteriole
4 terminal portal vein
5 portal canal - CT sheath surrounding the triad structures with periportal space (space of Mall)
6 sublobular vein
7 lymphatic vessel in the triad
8 arteriosinusoidal branch of the artery
9 bile ductule
10 inlet venule
11 hepatic sinusoid
12 central vein
13 liver parenchyma
14 bile canaliculi b/n each hepatocyte
15 openings of the sinusoids into the central veins
16 paraportal bile ductule (duct of Hering)
17 hepatocytes = liver parenchymal cells

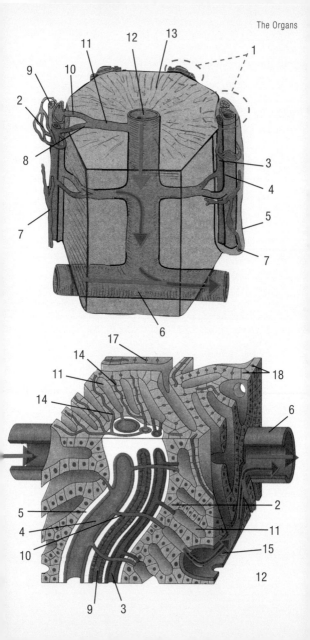

Liver

Micro Schema

Hepatocytes store glycogen, synthesize most of the plasma proteins, synthesize bile and detoxify the B & its cells. They have a high metabolic rate and are v sensitive to oxygen deprivation. They contain many mitos, ribosomes, peroxisomes and other vesicles.

1 endothelial cell are discontinuous along the sinusoid

2 space in the sinusoid b/n endothelial cells to allow the passage of large proteins

3 Küpffer cells are inserted into the sinusoidal lining and act like resident macrophages. They phagocytose worn out RBCs and FBs

4 reticular fibres - thin branched collagen fibre network to support the fragile parenchyma

5 bile canaliculus flanked by junctional complex (Jc) to prevent leakage of bile and facilitate bile secretion which is later collected in ductules

6 space of Disse, b/n the hepatocytes and the sinusoids

7 Ito cells - support the reticular fibres, a form of fibroblasts; in disease states these cells may store fat and produce many collagen fibres which interfere with the ability of material to diffuse b/n sinusoids & cells

8 mv border on 2 sides of the cell which face BVs

9 peroxisomes

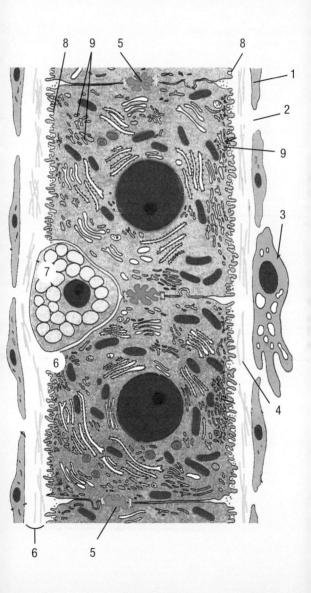

Lung

Macroscopic view

Anterior - in situ

Medial surfaces - removed and "opened" to show the inner surfaces

The lungs occupy most of the thoracic cavity, on either side of the heart. The pleural sacs wrap the lung parenchymal tissue and then coat the inner surface of the ribs and intercostal muscles as a double sac and it is the negative pressure generated by the rib cage expansion that draws air in. They are the site of oxygenation of the BF from the R side of the heart. The deoxygenated arterial blood comes in via the pulmonary arteries and the oxygenated venous blood leaves via the pulmonary veins and enters the LA. Organs and BVs passing through the thorax and leave impressions on the surface of these soft pliable organs.

1 cricoid cartilage
2 thyroid gld
3 L lung
   i = superior lobe
   ii = cardiac notch
   iii = inferior lobe
4 intercostal muscles
5 parietal pleural lining
6 oblique fissure b/n the 2 lobes
7 pericardium - enclosing the heart
8 thymus
9 diaphragm
   r =recess
10 R lung
   i = superior lobe
   ii = middle lobe
   iii = inferior lobe
11 first rib
12 trachea
13 root of the lung
14 pulmonary v
15 pulmonary a
16 main bronchus
17 hilar LNs = bronchopulmonary LNs

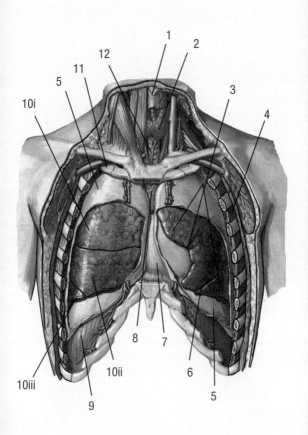

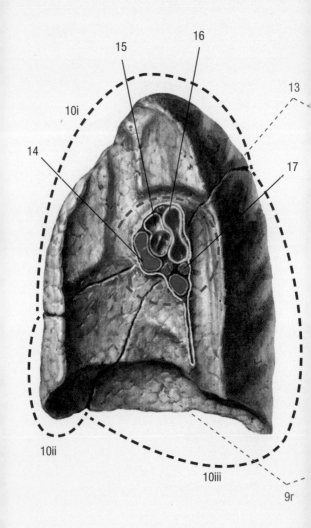

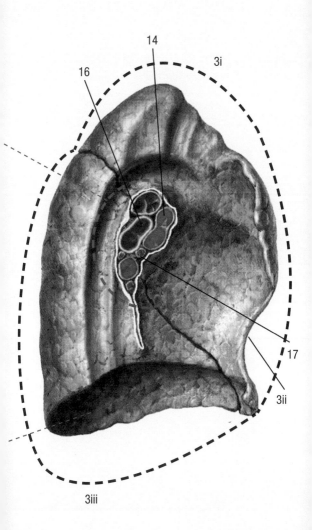

Lung

Macroscopic view
Larynx, Trachea & Bronchial tree

The lungs are the site of blood oxygenation, and the air must move through many air passages before they reach the site of gaseous exchange, beginning with oral and nasal cavities, larynx and trachea. Because the air is dragged in under negative pressure, these passages must remain open, and they do this via cartilage rings which are present until the level of the respiratory bronchioles. These are connected via inter-cartilage ligaments.

A Larynx

B Trachea

C Bronchial tree

1 Hyoid bone
2 thyroid cartligae
3 cricoid cartilage
4 tracheal cartilage
5 annular intercartilage lig
6 main bronchus
> L = left - more horizontal
> R = right - straighter - more likely to aspire food
7 L superior lobar bronchus
8 L superior segmental bronchus
9 L inferior lobar bronchus
10 tracheal carina = tracheal bifurcation
11 R segmental bronchus - this is the smallest anatomical unit of the lung
12 R middle lobar bronchus
13 median cricothyroid ligament

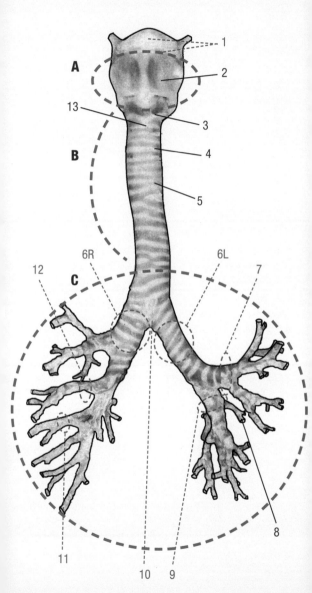

A

13

B

6R

6L

7

12

C

11

10

9

8

Lung

Histology

Transverse section LP H&E - overview showing most of the basic structures

The lung is a double-lined bag composed of a number of airways leading to thin walled closed sacs - the alveoli. It is here that the gases are exchanged along concentration lines - via slow flowing low P capillaries.

1. serosa = visceral peritoneum -
   c = inner layer of CT & BVs
   m = outer layer mesothelium
2. alveolar duct
3. respiratory bronchiole
4. alveolus - area of gas exchange
5. terminal bronchiole + pulmonary vein
6. pulmonary a & v
7. bronchial hyaline cartilage plates
8. bronchial glands with ducts
9. bronchus
10. pseudostratified epithelial lining with underlying mucosa
11. smooth m
12. submucosa
13. adventitia
14. lymphatic nodule
15. mucosal folds
16. trabeculae + BVs
17. alveolar sacs

Note 10, 12 & 13 are all composed of lamina propria

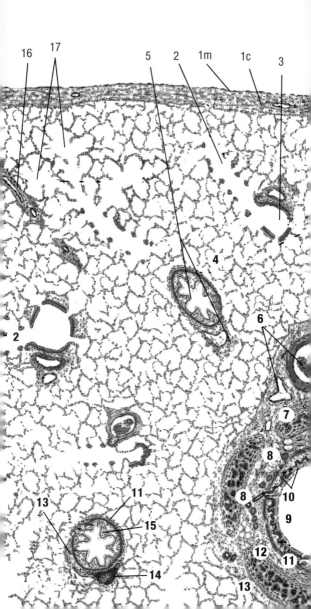

Lung
Respiratory passages

Histology

Transverse section through the passages of
MP intrapulmonary bronchus
HP terminal bronchiole

Air is transported from the outside to the alveoli via a series of passages which become smaller & smaller, while losing their wall thickness and structure progressively through the respiratory tree: commencing with the trachea → bronchi → bronchioles → alveolar sacs. Between the bronchi & the bronchioles cartilage is lost in the wall and the lining cells change from pseudostratified columnar epithelial cell to simple columnar cells.

1 alveoli
2 hyaline cartilage + epichondrium
3 pulmonary v
4 submucosal glands in the submucosa
5 mucosa
6 adipose T
7 pseudostratified columnar epithelium
8 pulmonary a containing B
9 serous glands + ducts
10 muscularis (smooth m)
11 columnar epithelium
12 LP - of the mucosa + submucosa

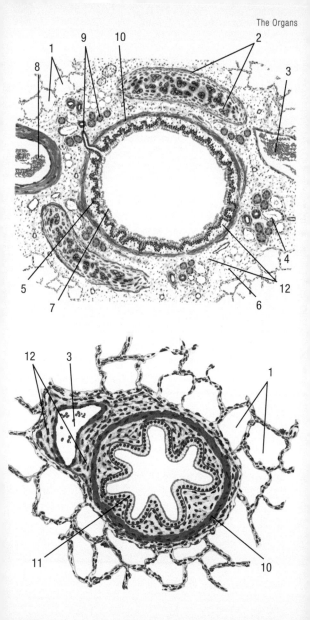

Lung
Linings & Alveoli

Histology
HP tracheal lining
HP alveoli

The lining of the passages is many cells thick and the main function is to make sure the air entering is dust free, warm & moist. The lining of the alveoli is very thin to allow for the exchange of O_2 and CO_2 and re-oxygenate the B.

1 demilune of the seromucous gld
2 serous gld
3 BM
4 pseudostratified columnar ciliated epithelium - this T changes with irritation to become truly stratified (e.g. with smokers)
5 cilia lining the trachea, these structures are lost with metaplasia of the epithelium
6 goblet cells
7 nuclear rows - note this is a simple epithelium - i.e. all the cells touch the BM & only the nuclei are multilayered
8 pulmonary v
9 duct of serous or mucus glds
10 pulmonary a
11 hyaline cartilage - part of the tracheal ring
12 perichondrium
13 type I pneumocyte
14 alveolar macrophage - dust cells
15 alveolar capillary
16 alveolar septum
17 smooth m in the terminal alveolar duct
18 type II pneumocyte
19 alveolar space

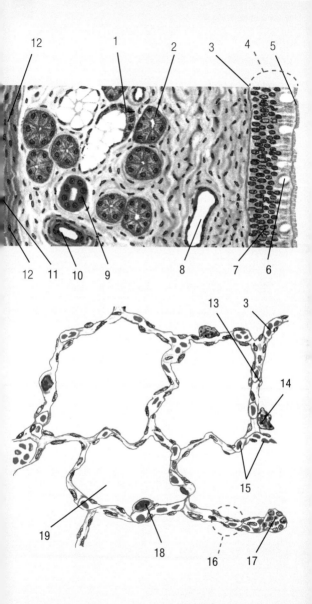

Lung
Air Blood Barrier

Schema

The site of gaseous exchange is the alveoli which have thin flattened walls covered in a flat endothelium, and thin walled capillaries which have fused BM.

Other cells present are resident macrophages, which destroy any small FBs which may be inhaled.

1   type II pneumocyte = resident macrophage
2   type I pneumocyte - endothelial cell
3   RBC in capillary
4   collagen & elastin fibres - essential for structure and recoil
5   alveolar pore - communication b/n 2 alveolar sacs
6   fibroblast - to support fibrillar components
7   fused BMs of capillary and alveolar walls

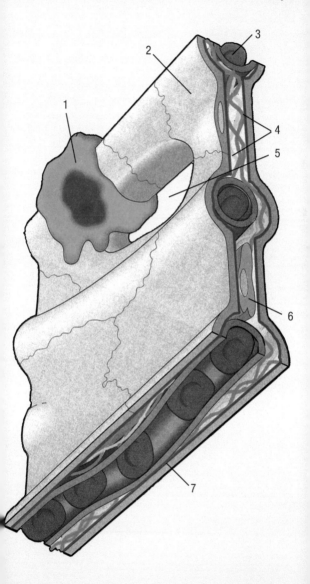

Lymph Node (LN)

Histology

LP H&E overview of whole structure

LNs are found throughout the body, generally flanking large BVs. They are small, beanlike structures connected via a series of interdigitating lymphatics. They return the leftover filtered fluid & proteins from the capillaries to the CVS after exposing them to their lymphatic T. Afferent lymphatics pierce the capsule; the plasma then flows through the subcapsular space and alongside the CT septae which carry lymphatics and hilar BVs. Triggers in the fluid may provoke the immune reaction, which causes the formation of germinal centres. It is then collected and leaves via efferent lymphatics and may return directly to the CVS or via another LN.

1 capsular adipose T - may be part of a mesentery
2 capsule & capsular BVs
3 hilum
4 efferent lymphatics
5 medullary cords
6 subcapsular space = marginal space
7 lymph nodules & the germinal centres (activated nodules)
8 arterioles & venules
9 CT septal vessels in CT septae (trabeculae)
10 afferent lymphatics
11 lymphocytes – loose lymphatic T

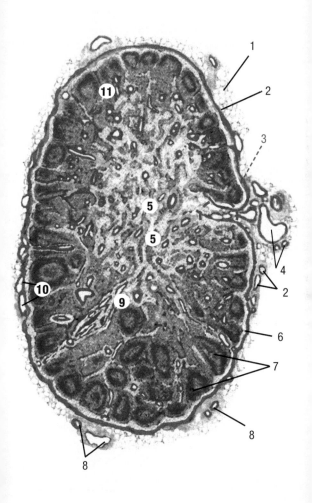

Lymph Node (LN)

Histology

MP H&E overview of the cortex & medulla
HP Mallory stain of the subcapsular sinus
HP reticular stain of the subcapsular sinus

Afferent lymphatics pierce the capsule of the LN; the plasma then flows through the subcapsular space and alongside the CT septae which carry lymphatics and hilar BVs. The many cell types present in the LN react to the plasma, determining the extent and type of immune &/or inflammatory response.

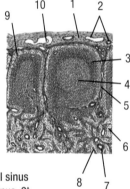

1 capsule
2 capsular BVs
3 cortical lymphoid nodules
4 germinal centre
5 CT trabecula containing BVs & lymphatics (5L)
6 medullary sinuses
7 medullary BVs
8 loose lymphoid T – in medullary cords
9 subcapsular sinus = marginal sinus continuous with trabecular sinus 9t
10 afferent lymphatics
11 reticular cells & fibres
12 lymphoblasts – lymphocytes capable of undergoing mitosis (12m)
13 macrophages
14 endothelial cell – discontinuous layer to enclose the lymphoid nodule

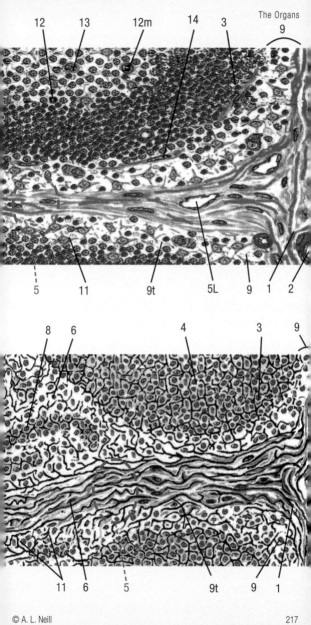

© A. L. Neill

Lymph Node (LN)

Schema

LNs are bean-shaped organs in a fibrous capsule. Lymph enters the LN and is exposed to the lymphocytes in the outer cortex, progresses through to the medulla and then out via the efferent lymphatics of the hilum, after which it goes to further LNs in the group or to the CVS, via the thoracic ducts. Lymphocytes also leave via the post-capillary venules. The venules are lined with tall endothelial cells which have receptors to attract lymphocytes and facilitate their transport out of the LN. If any of the entering material is antigenic it will trigger the start of the immune reaction.

1. hilum vessels - artery, vein & efferent lymphatic
2. medullary sinuses & loose cords of lymphocytes
3. capsule and subcapsular sinus
4. lymphatic nodules (follicles) ± active (germinal) centres of lymphocyte proliferation
5. dense lymphocytic tissue of the cortex
6. deep cortex = paracortex
7. CT trabecula - with surrounding sinus
8. afferent lymphatics & valve
9. capillary network
10. post-capillary (high endothelial) venules

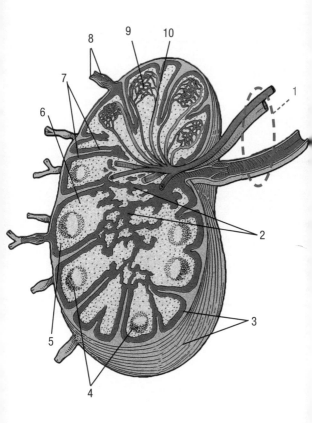

Pancreas

Macroscopic view
Anterior - with T cutaway to show the ducts entering
the duodenum

The pancreas is a grey comma-shaped organ up to 15cm long,
fixed to the posterior abdominal wall - lying in the upper abdomen
and extending from the R – where its head inserts into the "C" of the
duodenum – to the L where its tail extends into the hilum of
the spleen.

It is both an exocrine and endocrine gland. It produces digestive
enzymes. These are secreted via the serous glands into the pancreatic
duct which travels to the descending duodenum. It also produces Ns
into the BS most importantly insulin & glucagon from its endocrine
islets (islets of Langerhans).

1   common bile duct
2   tale of the pancreas
3   body of the pancreas
4   pancreatic duct
5   head of the pancreas
6   opening – common to the pancreatic duct and common
    bile duct –

      note this appears as a papilla in the mucosa of the
      duodenum = Duodenal papilla

7   pancreatic sphincter = sphincter of Oddi
      accessory pancreatic duct – present in 70%

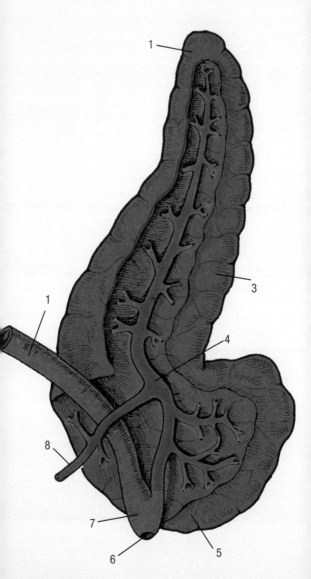

Pancreas

Histology
LP H&E overview

The pancreas is an organ with both an exocrine and endocrine gland, involved in digestion and sugar level balance, respectively. Examination shows the presence of Pacinian corpuscles which are pressure sensitive sensory receptors. Their function is unknown but it is speculated they may play a role in reporting on the state of the internal organ.

1   interlobular duct
2   Pacinian corpuscle - pressure sensitive receptor similar to that found in the skin and mesentery T
3   capillary through the glands
4   capillary in the endocrine pancreatic islets
5   Islet of Langerhan's - pancreatic islet - producing glucagon & insulin
6   serous cell - producing digestive enzymes
7   capillary b/n and around the serous glands not w/n them
8   interlobular septum of CT
9   interlobular BV

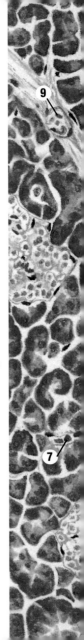

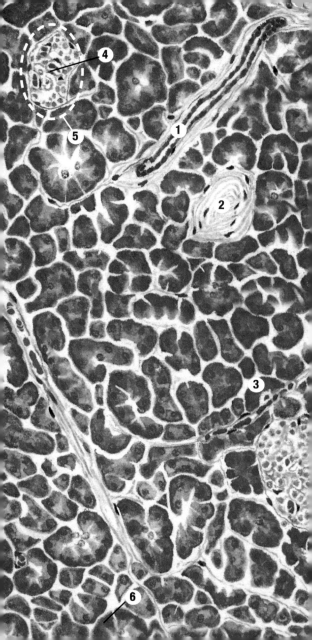

Pancreatic islets = Islets of Langerhans

Histology

HP to demonstrate the various cell types in the islets

The pancreas's endocrine component is the islets. There are at least 5 types of islet cells, which have specific H secretions.

1   serous cells - exocrine secretions
2   islet cells
3   intercalated duct
4   reticular fibrous network
5   α cells – 10-20% of islet cells - produce glucagon
6   β cells – 60-80% of islet cells - produce insulin & amylin
7   δ cells – 3-10% of islet cells - produce somatostatin
8   γ cells <3% of islet cells - producing pancreatic polypeptide
9   ε cells <1% of islet cells - produce ghrelin
10 fenestrated capillaries

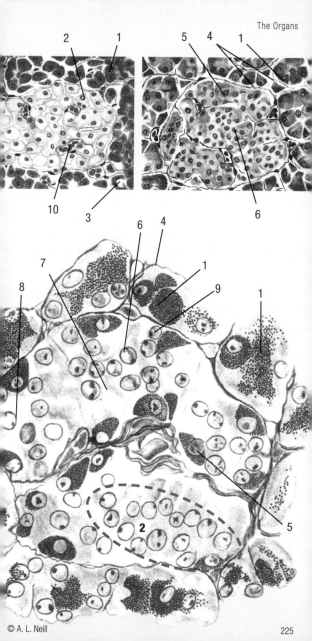

© A. L. Neill

Pancreas

Schema

The pancreas has small endocrine islets – islets of Langerhan's – sitting amidst serous exocrine glands which secrete digestive enzymes into the second part of the duodenum (descending duodenum). So it demonstrates the 2 forms of BS to these different gland types. The islets contain at least 4 different types of cells but the main cells types are the glucagon producing α cells (10-20%), which liberate glucose from the cells and the insulin producing β cells (60-80%), which allow entrance of sugars into the cells for use & storage. Somatostatin secreted by the δ cells regulate the use of sugar by affecting the α & β cells directly. The serous glands secrete enzymes in an alkaline solution to both digest the chyme from the stomach and to neutralize its acidity.

1 interlobular collecting duct
2 serous gland
3 acinar cell of the serous gland = exocrine gland
4 pancreatic islet = endocrine gland
    a = alpha cells
    b = beta cells
    v = capillaries b/n the islet cell
5 CT stroma = septum b/n the glands
6 intercalated ducts
7 a & v with capillaries traversing through the islets

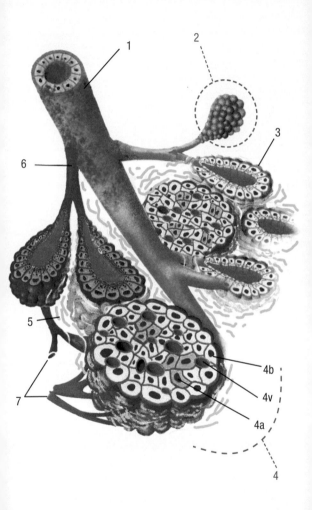

Pharynx - "throat"

Macro schema

Posterior - schema intact

Posterior - with divided constrictor muscles to show the interior of the "throat"

The pharynx is part of the throat - the area at the back of the mouth (12-15cm) which connects the mouth with the oesophagus and so it begins under voluntary control and then becomes automatic.

A = NASO-PHARYNX

B = ORO-PHARYNX

C = LARYNGO-PHARYNX

A+B+C = pharynx

1 Skull
2 adenoid tonsil
3 soft palate
4 phayngeal constrictors
   i = inf / m = middle /
   s = superior
5 epiglottis
6 laryngeal inlet
7 cricoid cartilage
8 oesophageal mucosa
   – continuous with oral
   mucosa
9 oesophagus
10 piriform fossa & opening
   to oesophagus

11 oral mucosa – continues
   throughout the pharynx
12 tonsil
13 uvula
14 orophayngeal isthmus
15 palato-pharyngeal fold
16 nasal choane =
   turbinates
17 nasal septum
18 thyroid gld
19 parathyroid glds
20 tracheal cartilage
21 thyoid

© A. L. Neill

Pituitary gland

Macroscopic view
development

The pituitary gland's anatomy is often confusing mainly because of its complicated development. It is a fusion of the pharyngeal ectoderm adenohypophysis = the anterior lobe and the downgrowth of the neuroectoderm from the brain the neurohypophysis = the posterior lobe and the mass in b/n the middle lobe. There are 4 tropic - growth promoting - Hs from the ant. lobe: adrenocorticotropic hormone (ACTH), follicle stimulating hormone (FSH), luteinizing hormone (LH) & thyroid stimulating hormone (TSH), and these affect all the endocrine organs of the body either directly or indirectly.

1 supraoptic nucleus
2 optic chiasma
3 pars tuberalis
4 hypothalamohypophyseal tract
5 pars distalis = anterior lobe = adenohypohysis
      e = developed from the oropharynx ectoderm
6 follicles filled with colloid in the middle lobe
7 pars intermedia = middle lobe
8 pars nervosa = posterior lobe = neurohypophysis
      e = developed from the neuroectoderm
9 infundibulum
10 median eminence
11 paraventricular nucleus
12 sella turcica in the Sphenoid bone houses the
   pituitary securely
      e = from the developing sphenoid bone

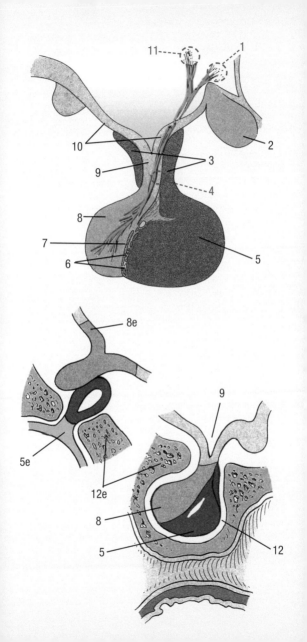

Pituitary gland

Histology
LP H&E overview with Azan staining HP inserts

The pituitary "gland" is a combination endocrine gland derived from the palate - adenohypophysis (the anterior lobe) & a down-growth of the brain's neural material - neurohypophysis (the posterior lobe).

1 pars tuberalis - stalk of the pituitary
2 pars intermedia - site of junction b/n the ant. & post. lobes - containing colloid material (c) in follicles
3 pars nervosa - posterior lobe - containing pituicytes (p)
4 veins in the capsule (around both lobes)
5 CT septa
6 capsule
7 sinusoidal capillaries - open - to allow for flow of large H molecules
8 pars distalis - ant lobe contains a number of specialized cells - with specific staining affinities - which are found throughout the lobe

    a = acidophils = α cells

    b = basophils = β cells

    c = chromophobes (colour haters)

9 infundibulum - funnel down into the gld from the brain ventricles

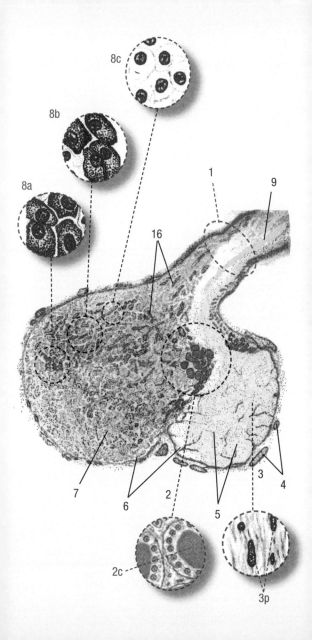

Pituitary gland

Schema - BS

The pituitary gland's endocrine functions are stimulated by the hypophyseal portal vein circulation (9, 4) and part of the hypothalamic endocrine axis. The 4 tropic - growth promoting - Hs of the anterior lobe are: adrenocorticotropic hormone (ACTH), follicle stimulating hormone (FSH), luteinizing hormone (LH) & thyroid stimulating hormone (TSH), affect all the endocrine organs of the body either directly or indirectly.

1   internal carotid a
2   superior hypophyseal a
3   hypophyseal portal v
4   hypophyseal v
5   secondary plexus - sinusoidal capillaries in the ant lobe
6   inferior hypophyseal a & v
7   middle lobe = pars intermedia
8   infundibulum
9   primary plexus - sinusoidal capillaries of the hypothalamus

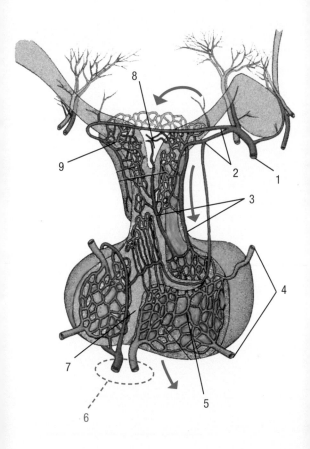

Salivary glands

Macroscopic view

There are 3 salivary glands named for their position in the mouth. The sublingual & submandibular glds have 2 types of exocrine glds in their structure in approx equal proportions – mucous & serous glds, whereas the parotid, the biggest gld, is mainly serous. It is only the content of the cells which vary, either they secrete mucous to lubricate the food, or amylase to begin digestion. In both cases the saliva produced is dilute and concentrated as it travels down the ducts. This allows, when eating a large amount of dilute saliva to assist in the process, but conserves fluid and helps to disinfect the mouth when resting, as amylase also has disinfectant properties.

1 frenulum of tongue
2 parotid duct
3 parotid gland a = accessory gland present in 50%
4 submandibular gld
5 submandibular duct
6 sublingual gld
7 sublingual ducts
8 opening of the submandibular ducts
9 collecting ducts of the glds
10 duct lumen
11 acina of the glds with saliva which is concentrated as it travels in the collecting ducts
12 acinar cells
13 tubular cells which concentrates the saliva as it travels down the duct

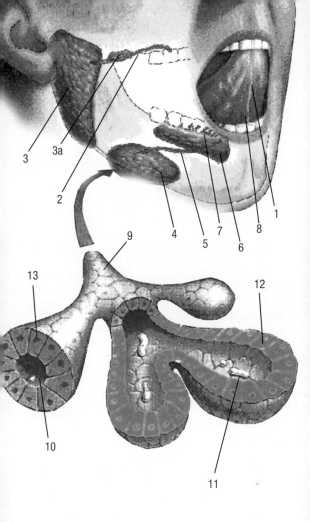

Salivary glands

Histology
Submandibular gland H&E MP with HP inserts

The submandibular gland has 2 types of glands present in approximately equal proportions serous and mucinous, the first begins the digestive process and the other helps in lubricating the food in preparation for swallowing.

1 serous gland - with secretory granules (g)

2 mucinous gland
   m = myoepithelial cell

3 intercalated duct

4 striated duct
   b = basal striations

5 adipose cells in the gland

6 interlobular excretory ducts - join to form larger ducts

7 serous demilune

8 interlobular CT septa with BVs

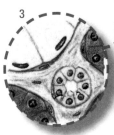

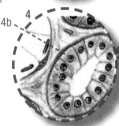

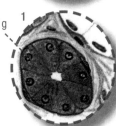

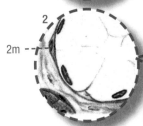

© A. L. Neill

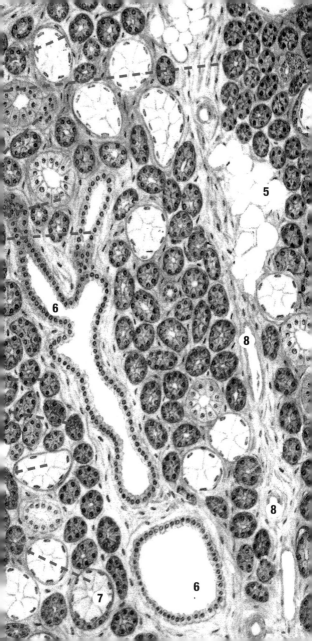

Salivary glands

Schema
Salivary glands proportions of gland types

The 3 main salivary glands have different proportions of serious and mucinous glands as demonstrated..

A = parotid

B = submandibular

C = sublingual

1   acini cells
   m = mucinous
   s = serous
2   intercalated duct
3   striated duct
4   excretory duct

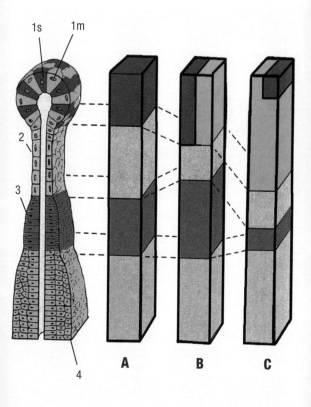

Skin
Hair follicle = Pilosebaceous unit

Macroscopic view

The hair follicle is a complex organ, involving several tissues working in cooperation and present on nearly all parts of the skin. There are about 5 million hair follicles on the human body even though most of them do not appear to have a useful function. They are greatly influenced by hormonal changes, life stressors and environmental factors. They are always associated with the acne and many other skin infections. The follicle basically is an epidermal structure similar to the nail, but has input from the dermal papilla, which determines its growth phases including extrusion and replacement.

1 hair
   - c = cuticle
   - m = medulla
   - o = cortex
   - s = shaft
2 epidermis
   - e = external root sheath (AKA outer root sheath)
   - i = internal root sheath (AKA inner root sheath)
3 dermis
4 apocrine sweat gland - associated with 2° sexual features
5 BM - extends to the base of the hair root
6 matrix
7 dermal papilla - supplies B to the hair
8 BVs to the hair papilla
9 sebaceous gld
10 sweat gld - eccrine
11 erector pili - skeletal m

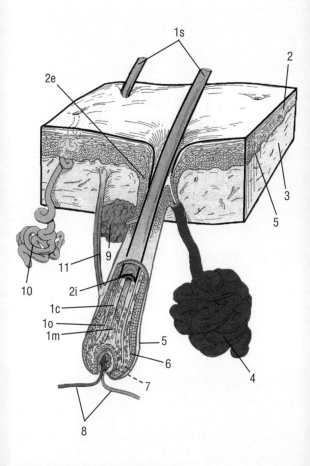

1s

2e

2

3

5

10

11

9

2i

1c

1o

1m

5

6

4

7

8

Skin
Hair follicle = pilosebaceous unit

Histology
LP H&E overview of the structure

All regions of the skin grow hair of one sort or another, except the thick skin of the soles and palms. The main differences are the length of the hair and the number & type of sebaceous glands associated with it. This very complex unit is actually an adnexa of the skin - even though it resides in the dermis. The CT and epithelium interact and both are needed to maintain the unit.

1 cortex - keratinized cells of the hair

2 cuticle

3 inner hair root sheath

4 outer hair root sheath

5 CT sheath

6 lymphatics + capillaries

7 hair matrix

8 hair bulb

9 capillaries of the dermal papilla

   m = melanin pigment in papilla

10 sweat gland

11 excretory ducts of the sweat gland

12 dermal CT

13 erector papillae m

14 sebaceous gland

   b = basal cells, d = duct

   e = degenerating cells added to the secretion - apocrine excretory duct

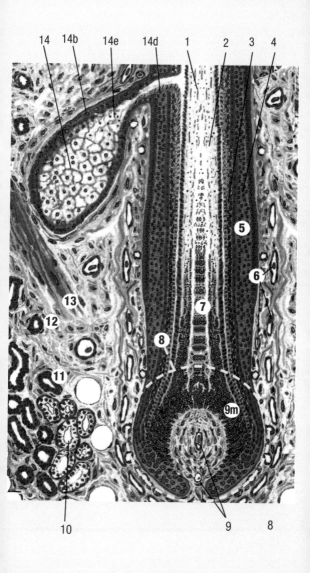

© A. L. Neill

Nails

Macroscopic view
Sagittal section

The nails are adnexae of the skin epithelium, like hair and they are made up of keratin the protein which forms the waterproof barrier of the skin and the shaft of the hair. The rate of nail growth depends upon the length of the distal phalanges.

1 body of the nail = nail plate
2 nail moon = lunula
3c cuticle = eponychium
3e free edge of the cuticle = perionyx
4 nail sinus
5 nail root = germinal matrix = onychostroma
6 epidermis
7 dermis
8 subcutaneous T / fat
9 distal phalange
10 quick = hyponychium
11 nail bed
12 free edge of the nail = margo liber
13 joint capsule & surrounding ligaments

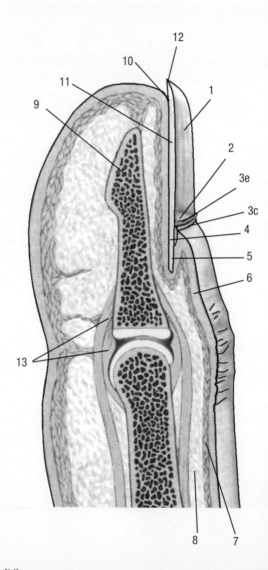

Skin
Finger tip - thick hairless skin

Histology + Macroscopic view

A fingertip showing rete ridges - for very firm epidermal binding

B LP Azan stain showing fibrous extensions into deep subcutaneous T

The skin varies significantly in different regions adapting to its environment. The fingertip sole and heel are all examples of thick hairless skin, and all have strong epithelial attachments and deep reticular dermis.

1 epidermis
2 dermis
3 subcutaneous T
4 CT septum
5 adipose T
6 BVs of the skin
7 sweat glands & ducts
8 reticular fibres of the reticular dermis
9 dermal papillae - invaginate into the epidermis and tightly bind it

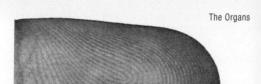

A

B

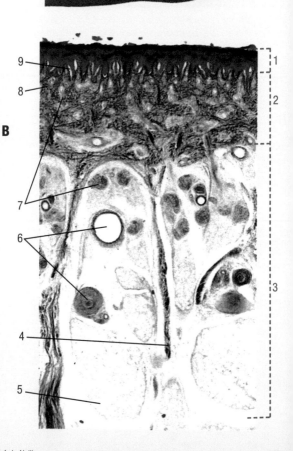

9
8

7

6

4

5

1
2

3

Skin
Thick hairless skin - dermal specializations

Histology

A Glomus bodies HP H&E

B Pacinian corpuscles H&E MP

Thick skin has a number of specialties in the dermis - present due to the function of these areas - Pacinian corpuscles to measure the pressure in the area and glomus bodies to facilitate BF and regulate the temperature.

1 sweat gld

    d = duct

    i = intercalated duct

    m= myoepithelial cell

    s = secreting portion

2 N from ANS - sympathetic

3 glomus body (AKA glomus apparatus)

4 AV shunt of the glomus to direct B either away or to the surface

5 venule

6 CT stroma of the dermis

7 adipose T

8 Pacinian corpuscle

    a =central axon

    c = CT capsule

    L = lamellae

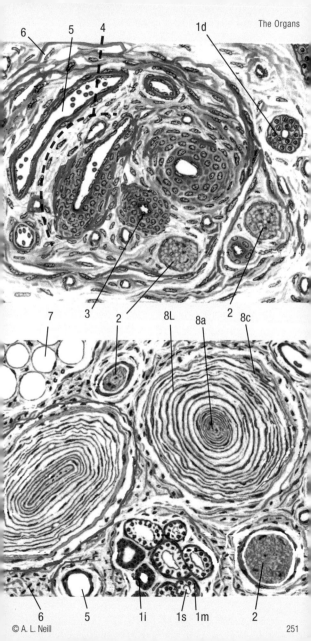

© A. L. Neill

Skin
Lip

Histology
MP H&E showing transition b/n thin hairy skin and mucous membranes (mm) of the the oral cavity

The skin varies significantly in different region adapting to its environment. The lip is a complex region – it has to be mobile and waterproof but changes quickly to the non-keratinized mm of the mouth where it is exposed to digestive enzymes of saliva.

1   sweat gld
2   erector pili m
3   sloughed off skin cells
4   stratified keratinized skin - of the outer lip
5   hair follicle
6   sebaceous glds
7   transition zone
8   orbicularis oris m
9   adipose T = fat cells
10   mm – of the oral cavity
11   mucous secreting labial glds

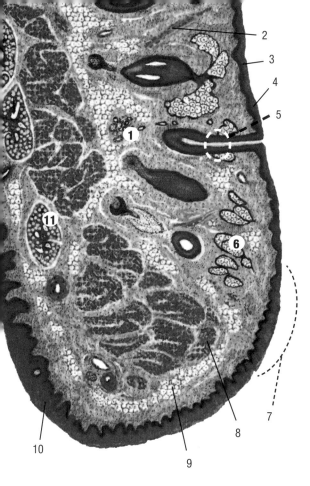

2

3

4

5

1

11

6

8

7

10

9

Spleen

Macroscopic view
Lateral view - anterior surface

The spleen occupies the LUQ, pressed up against the diaphragm. It is generally covered by ribs 9-11 but may extend deep into the abdominal space in disease, particularly parasitic diseases. It is a soggy bag of blood with a fragile capsule so that if exposed due to splenomegaly, it may be easily injured and bleed into the abdominal cavity.

1   margins of the spleen i = inferior / s = superior
2   gastrolienal lig
3   gastroepiploic a & v
4   tail of the pancreas
5   splenic neurovascular bundle
      a & v + lymphatic vessel, LN & splenic N
6   splenic recess - leading into the hilum of the spleen
7   short gastric a & v

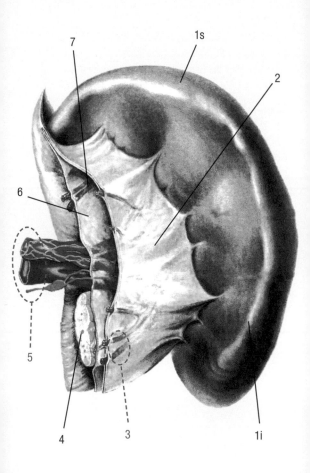

1s

7

2

6

5

4

3

1i

Spleen

Histology
LP overview showing tissue variations with HP inserts

The spleen is a large filter combining the functions of the liver & LNs. This organ cleans the blood - ridding it of all misshapen & old RBCs. It exposes Ags in the B to Abs on lymphocytes or phagocytosis by the many macrophages in the spleen and allows for an immune reaction to develop. When cut the surface appears as a soggy red bag (red pulp) - containing loose large capillaries flanked by macrophages and firmer white spots - the white pulp, containing large populations of lymphocytes.

1. splenic CT trabeculae
2. splenic capsule
3. RED PULP - filled with...
    - s = venous sinusoids
    - p = pulp arteries
4. WHITE PULP containing
    - c = central vein
    - g = germinal centre - of proliferating lymphocytes
    - L = lymphatic nodule

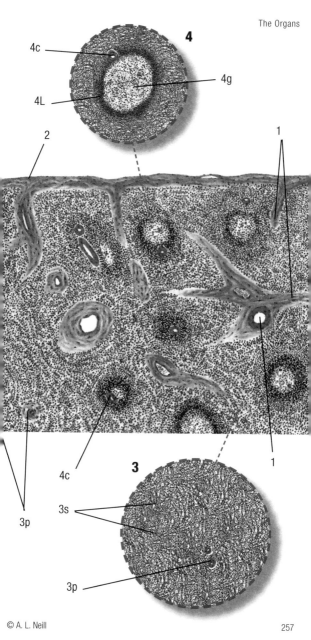

© A. L. Neill

Spleen

Schema
open and closed circulation in detail
The circulation of the spleen has 2 forms:

arteriole → nothing the open circulation - (O)

RBCs are free in the parenchyma and the sinus venules where endothelial cells are removed and collagen coils loosely hold the blood cells with macrophages flanking the vessel and "tasting" the cells inside to determine any (inflammatory or immune response) closed (C).

1   endothelial lining
2   BM
3   macrophages
4   RBCs
5   venous sinus
6   collagen coils

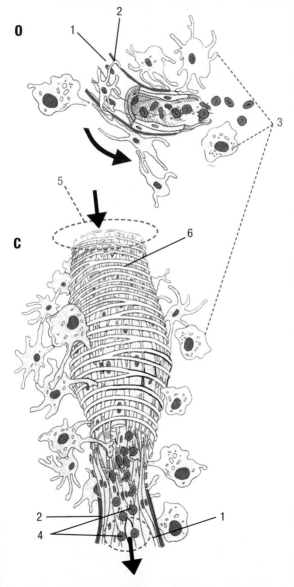

0

C

Stomach
Regional Variations

Schema

The stomach has distinct overlapping regions with a different mixture and proportion of glands designed protect the organ from its own acid secretions. With age more cells produce acid and the mucosa is less protected. Due to the closeness to the heart, pain from the oesophagus and upper region of the stomach are often indistinguishable.

1   oesophagus

2   cardiac region = cardia - the region most at risk from acid erosion

3   b = body / f = fundus - same regions anatomically except that the fundal region is involved in hiatus hernia and often contains gas

4   pyloris s = sphincter - region most protected from acid erosion

5   duodenum

6   mucosa

7   muscularis mucosa

8   glands

> b = base - producing acid and enzyme
>
> n = neck - transition section where stem cells and mitotic figures are found
>
> s = superficial - producing mucous layer to protect the stomach lining

    © A. L. Neill

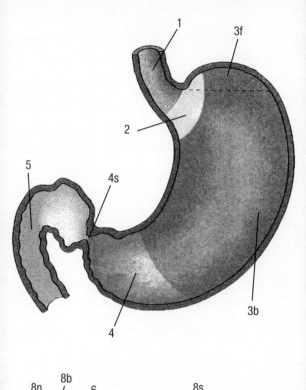

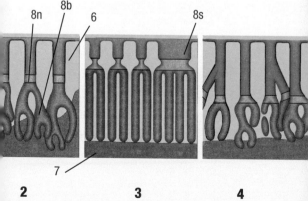

2   **3**   **4**

Thymus

Macroscopic view
Anterior

The thymus is a small insignificant organ in the anterior mediastinum. In the child it is much larger and plays a significant role in the child's developing immunity, but it degenerates with age.

1   L lung
2   L lobe of the thymus
3   anterior surface of the pericardium
4   body of the thymus
5   SVC
6   Brachial plexus

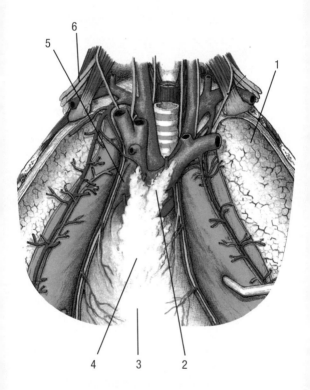

Thymus

Histology
LP HP overview H&E showing the main tissue structure and layout

The thymus (20-30gms) is found in the anterior mediastinum. It is lobular with CT trabeculae. Lymphocytes transported from the bone marrow are differentiated into T lymphocytes here. These further differentiate and move to other organs, particularly LNs. With age the fat cells replace the immune cells until the thymus is relatively depleted of immune cells in the adult.

1 adipose cells in the trabeculae
2 BVs in the trabeculae
3 capsule
4 arteriole
5 fat cells in the cortex - with age these increase
6 medulla + thymic corpuscle (= Hassell's corpuscle)*
7 cortex
8 lobule
9 epithelial reticular cells in medulla
10 T lymphocytes

the role of the corpuscle is unknown - it consists of flattened epithelial cells with a degenerative centre, and is only found in thymic T.

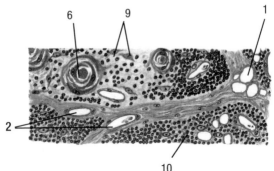

© A. L. Neill

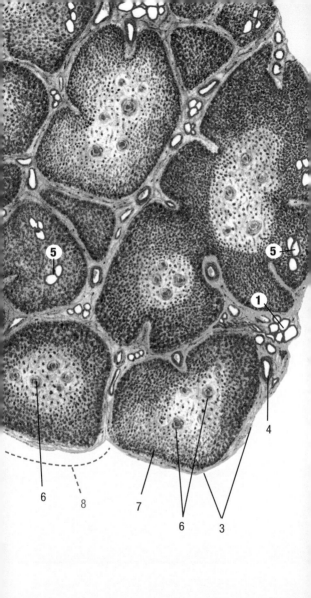

Thyroid gland

Macroscopic view
Anterior
Posterior

The thyroid gland is encapsulated and straddles the trachea at T1. It has 2 lobes and a connecting isthmus as well as occasionally an additional pyramidal lobe which lies along and up the trachea. The post. surface encloses the 4 parathyroid glands but their functions are not related.

1   thyroid cartilage
2   cricoid cartilage - site of the pyramidal lobe if present
3   isthmus
4   inferior parathyroid gland + lower pole of the thyroid
5   body of thyroid - lobe
6   upper pole of the thyroid
7   inferior constrictor of the pharynx
8   post surface of the thyroid
9   superior parathyroid gland
10 oesophagus
11 transition b/n pharynx and oesophagus - Killen's triangle

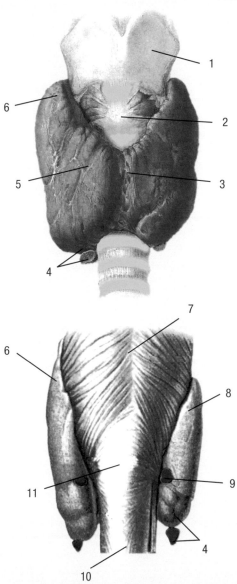

Thyroid gland

Macroscopic view
Transverse in 2 planes - higfher C6, lower T1

The thyroid gland is encapsulated and straddles the trachea at T1. It has 2 lobes and a connecting isthmus as well as occasionally an additional pyramidal lobe, which lies along and up the trachea.

1. thyroid parenchyma with CT septa
2. tracheal fascia
3. isthmus - showing cut surface & superior edge
4. superior a & v
5. anterior surface of the L lobe
6. middle cervical fascia = pretracheal fascia
7. superior pole of R lobe
8. internal jugular v
9. common carotid a
10. prevertebral fascia
11. trachea
12. T1 vertebral body
13. oesophagus
14. L recurrent laryngeal N
15. L Vagus N

T1

8

6

7

5

9

10

4

11

12

3

2

14

13

1

15

C6

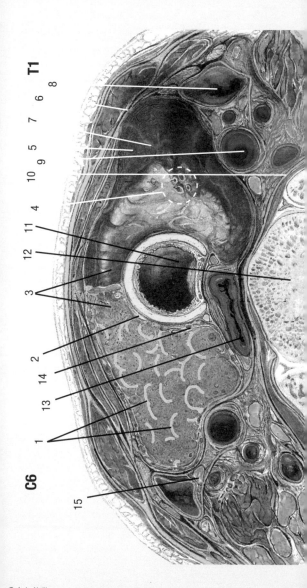

Thyroid gland
& Parathyroid gland

Histology

LP

HP

The thyroid gland is encapsulated and straddles the trachea. It consists of many follicles which store the H in an inactive state bound to colloid. A single epithelial layer lines the follicles, sitting on a BM and surrounded by BVs. Follicles in various stages of activity can be found throughout the gland.

The parathyroid gland abuts the posterior surface of the thyroid sharing the capsule, but has an independent function.

1 capsule and CT septum
2 colloid in the follicles
3 mv border on the apex of the lining cells
4 lining epithelial cells - cuboidal but may be columnar when active
5 parafollicular cells
6 venule
7 capillary
8 CT septum of the parathyroid gld
9 oxyphil cells of the parathyroid gld
10 chief cells of the parathyroid gld

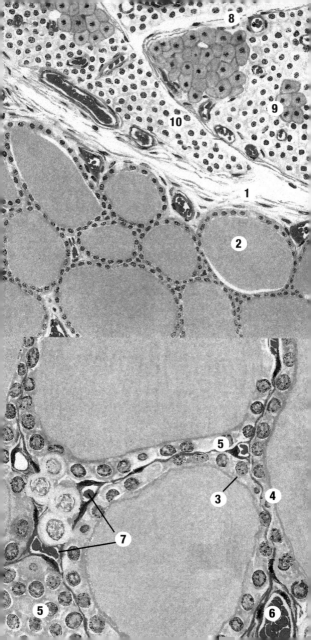

Thyroid gland

Schema

A Synthesizing cell

B Resting cell

C Secreting cell

The thyroid gland synthesizes, stores & releases thyroid Hs (T3 & T4), and these activities may all be occurring at once w/in the thyroid gland. Although an endocrine gland the H secretion is stored ec and must be retrieved via pseudopodal resorption before release.

1. AAs in the BV - absorbed into the cell
2. go to rER for synthesis of thyroglobulin + peroxidase
3. go to Golgi for added sugars
4. release of thyroglobulin + peroxidase into the follicle
5. iodide absorbed from the BS
6. released and converted to iodine by peroxidase in the follicle
7. formation of the thyroid Hs T3 & T4 - which then combine with the colloid
8. colloid storage material
9. mv - range in size depending upon the function of the cell - longer when active
10. Jc in the cell - to prevent passage of material b/n the cells
11. large numbers of mitos when cell is active
12. pseudopod - to phagocytose large colloid droplets
13. combination colloid + H
14. lysosome - which combines with phagosome and liberates the Hs - T3 & T4
15. release of Hs directly into the BV
16. BM - of gland and BVs
17. capillary lumen

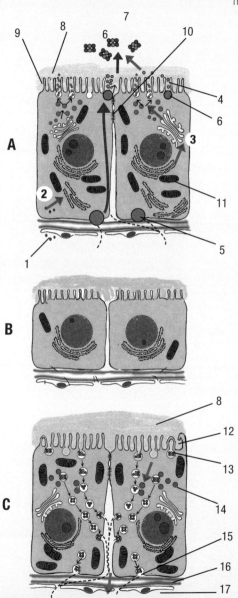

© A. L. Neill

Tongue

Macroscopic view
Dorsal surface

The tongue is one of the strongest muscles in the body covered with a non-keratinized stratified epithelium. Inserted into this organ are specialist structures the tastebuds along with mucous glands and its posterior border is made up of tonsilar lymphoid tissue.

1 Epiglottis
2 median glossoepiglottic fold
3 epiglottic vallecula – crevice
4 root of the tongue - posterior 1/3 – immobile part of the tongue
5 palatopharyngeus
6 palatine tonsil
7 palatoglossus
8 triangular fold
9 palatoglossal arch
10 median sulcus
11 dorsum of the tongue – pre-sulcus
12 margin of the tongue
13 body
14 tip of tongue = apex

15 site of filiform papillae
16 fungiform papillae
17 folate papillae
18 circumvallate papillae
19 dorsum of the tongue – post-sulcus
20 sulcus terminalis
21 tonsilar fossa & crypts
22 foramen caecum
23 lingual tonsils – on the root / base of the tongue
24 lateral glossoepiglottic fold

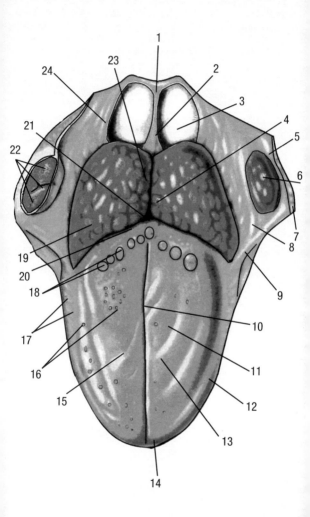

Tongue

Histology
LP H&E overview of the tip of the tongue dorsal (A) and ventral (B) surfaces
MP H&E circumvallate papillae - base of the tongue dorsal surface
HP H&E taste buds in situ

The tongue tip has several functions including taste and speech. Due to this it has many skeletal muscle and CT insertions in various planes allowing for multi-directional movement. It is highly vascularized with mucous and serous acini in the sublingual salivary glands.

The distal region has the smaller fungiform filiform papillae which have embedded taste buds, the circumvallate papillae are found further back - distal to the lingual tonsils, and the last papillae found on the tongue.

1 filiform & fungiform papillae with taste buds
2 skeletal m - various planes
3 venule
4 collected excretory duct of the sublingual gland
5 ant. lingual salivary gland with serous & mucous acini and intercalated excretory ducts
6 N cells
7 stratified squamous epithelium
8 artery
9 LP
10 CT trabeculae with BVs
11 taste bud
12 serous acini
13 excretory ducts
14 lymphatics + capillaries
15 furrow b/n papillae = crypts
16 taste pore with mv - taste hairs
17 sloughed off cells from the epithelium
18 gustatory cell = taste cells - associated with N fibres
19 basal cells
20 sustenacular cell = supporting cells

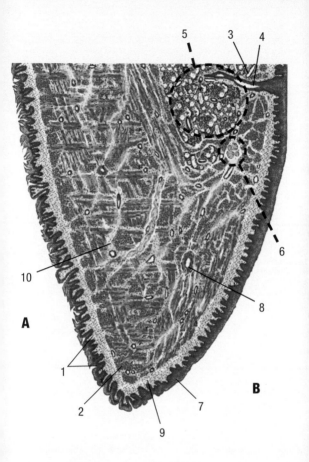

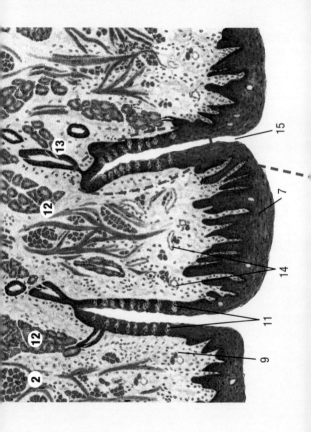

© A. L. Neill

11

14

20

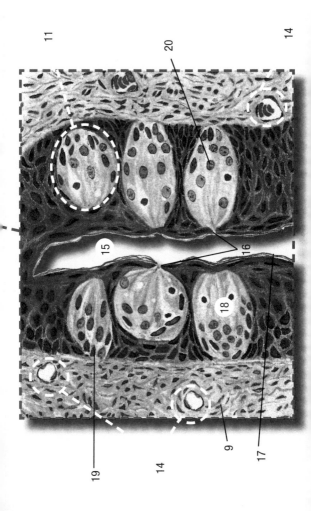

15

16

18

19

14

9

17

Tongue - taste bud

Micro Schema

The taste bud is a mini organ - w/n the major organ of the tongue. Taste buds are found throughout the tongue's dorsal surface concentrated at the tongue's base but more distal than the tonsil and embedded deep in the crypts of the papillae.

1   taste pore
2   mv
3   supporting cells = sustenacular cells
4   basal cell = mitosing cells found here
5   taste cell special sensory – only one modality to each cell
6   sensory N fibres synapse onto the surface of the cell and directly interact
7   N fibres around the taste bud – afferent – not special sensory
8   stratified non-keratinized epithelium
9   BM

Areas on the tongue detect certain tastes more sensitively although it is now thought that this is more flexible, and all areas have sensitivity to all forms of taste, one cell at a time.

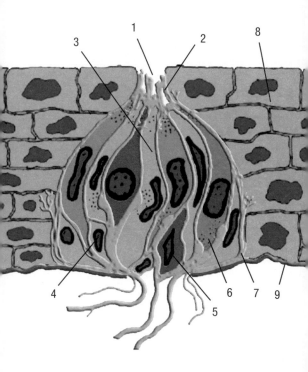

Tonsils

Histology
A Lingual LP H&E overview
B Palatine LP H&E overview

Tonsils are collections of lymphoid tissue placed in strategic places in the mouth and pharynx. Large in children, they can swell and impede breathing and swallowing, when they stimulated in the immune reaction and for this reason are often removed. They shrink in the adult and may become scarred and fibrous. Lingual tonsils are placed at the back of the tongue further back than the taste buds and covered in stratified epithelium.

1 stratified epithelium (non-keratinized)
2 lymphoid tissue
3 germinal centre in lymphoid nodule capsule
4 LP
5 mucous acini of the posterior mucous glands
6 skeletal m of the tongue
7 adipose cells
8 exocrine gland excretory ducts
9 tonsil
10 tonsilar crypts
11 CT trabecula with BVs
12 CT capsule

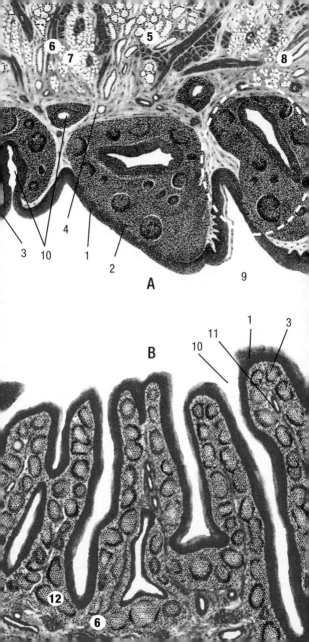

Notes